D1437207
305984062.

THE BASIC NEUROLOGY OF SPEECH

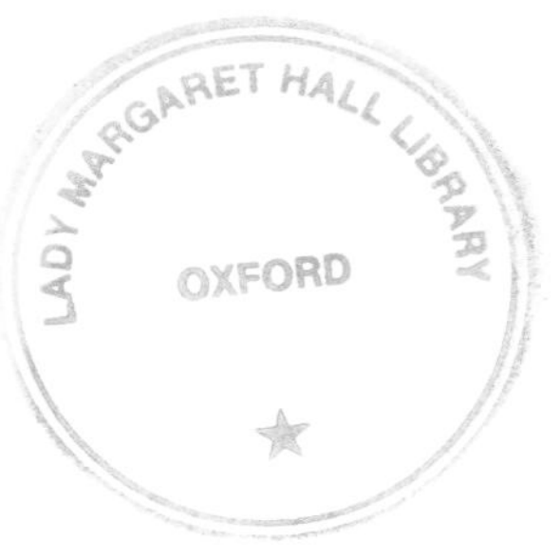

THE BASIC NEUROLOGY OF SPEECH

MICHAEL L. E. ESPIR

M.A., M.B., M.R.C.P.

*Consultant Neurologist, Nottingham University Hospital Group and Regional Department of Neurosurgery and Neurology, Derbyshire Royal Infirmary.
Examiner in Neurology, College of Speech Therapists.
Formerly lecturer in Neurology, Oldrey-Fleming and Leicester Schools of Speech Therapy.*

AND

F. CLIFFORD ROSE

M.B., M.R.C.P., D.C.H.

*Consultant Physician in Neurology Charing Cross and West London Hospitals, Consultant Neurologist Moor House School for Speech Disorders, Oxted, and John Horniman School, Worthing. Member of the Examinations Board, College of Speech Therapists.
Examiner in Neurology for B.Sc. (Speech), University of Newcastle upon Tyne.
Formerly lecturer in Neurology, Oldrey-Fleming and Central Hospital Schools of Speech Therapy.*

BLACKWELL SCIENTIFIC PUBLICATIONS
OXFORD AND EDINBURGH

SBN 632 07500 7

FIRST PUBLISHED 1970

Printed in Great Britain by

THE SALISBURY PRESS

and bound by

THE KEMP HALL BINDERY

CONTENTS

PREFACE

There is a vast literature on the many disciplines with which speech is concerned, but this book is intended as a simple presentation of the neurological approach to its anatomy, physiology and pathology. Although based on courses of lectures given by the authors in three of the schools of speech therapy in Great Britain, it should prove helpful not only to speech therapists, both for their final examinations and for practice afterwards, but also to medical students and others in disciplines concerned with communication, e.g. paediatrics, psychiatry, psychology, phonetics and linguistics.

The neurological mechanisms of speech and its disorders are complex and because of our pragmatic simplification a selected bibliography is given.

It is a pleasure to acknowledge our indebtedness to our teachers and colleagues who are too numerous to mention individually. We are particularly grateful to Professor W. Ritchie Russell and the Clarendon Press for permission to quote from the book *Traumatic Aphasia*, and also to Dr. Macdonald Critchley and the late Lord Brain for their teaching and literature.

We also thank the authors and publishers who have given permission for the reproduction of the illustrations acknowledged in the text. We are grateful to Dr. Paul Millac for reading the proofs and making helpful suggestions, and to Mr B. Armitage, Librarian at the Charing Cross Hospital Medical School for preparing the index.

Our thanks are due to Mrs Vanessa Dussek and Mrs Patricia Espir for their patience in typing and retyping the chapters, and to the Department of Medical Illustration of Charing Cross Hospital for help with diagrams.

CHAPTER 1

INTRODUCTION

Speech is unique to man. It can be defined as a system of communication in which thoughts are expressed and understood by using acoustic symbols. They are produced by the vibration of the vocal cords in the larynx (phonation), caused by the flow of air (respiration) and given final form by movements of the lips, tongue and palate (articulation).

Speech refers to verbal symbols, but language includes the non-verbal aspects of communication, for example—gesticulation, gesture and pantomime, each of which is different. Gesticulation is the associated muscular movement which emphasises speech. Pantomime is a method of communication in which spoken language is replaced by acting, and may include a series of gestures, each of which conveys a single meaning. Language includes all systems of communication, not only speech but the expression and understanding of written words, signs, gestures and music.

THE DEVELOPMENT OF SPEECH

It is important to realise firstly the comparatively late acquirement of speech in biological history (phylogenetic development), and secondly to understand how an individual person learns to speak (ontogenetic development).

Phylogenetic Development

The age of the planet on which we live has been estimated as 2000 million years. Life in its earliest form occurred in about half that time, i.e. 1000 million years. An animal capable of making a noise (i.e. possessing a jointed larynx) came into existence 200 million years ago, but true and false vocal cords with the formation of a cochlea did not take place until perhaps 50 million years ago.

Although some animals, for example, the cock, hawk and rat make signals, and apes chatter and lions roar, these sounds are inborn, species-characteristic and limited to a specific reaction. The talking of parrots is mimicry and not speech in the scientific sense since there is no question of the bird formulating thoughts into words or understanding the sounds it utters. The 'language' of birds is in fact limited to communicating their desire for food, sexual needs, warnings of danger or mimicry, whereas human language covers an infinite number of thoughts, abstract as well as concrete. Questions can be asked and answered allowing an exchange of ideas and arguments and humans also have the unique privilege of telling lies, believing or disbelieving. Although the faculty of speech is inborn, individual language has to be learnt.

There are several hypotheses as to how man acquired speech. Max Müller described the following: (1) the 'Ding-dong' theory—suggesting that there is an inherent connection between words and the things they stand for; (2) the 'Bow-wow' theory—suggesting that speech arose out of onomatopoetic sounds; (3) the 'Pooh-pooh' theory indicating that by involuntary sounds, and interjection, speech was acquired; like the 'speech' of lower animals and birds; and (4) the 'Yo-heave-ho' theory—suggesting that man began to learn to speak from the sounds associated with communal physical effort. Early speech consisted of cries of emotion, e.g. fear, joy, anger and these corresponded to animal sound signals. Curses and exclamations lack the distinctive features of human speech since they may be uttered involuntarily and are automatic expressions of the emotions. Some of these interjections are conventially described as 'whew', 'ah', 'urgh', humph'.

The earliest man of which we have evidence (Java man) lived about one million years ago. A more developed creature (Heidelberg man) appeared half a million years ago, Neaderthal man about 150,000 years ago, and Cromagnon man about 50,000 years ago. Man began to speak as soon as he used tools, (i.e. during the first Pleistocene period): the cooperation of individuals is needed both for speech and the use of tools and probably the first role of speech was to control behaviour.

Man did not give up his nomadic life and develop agriculture until 7000 B.C., whereas the first writing of which we have evidence is approximately 4000 B.C.: the Samarians of Mesopotamia were writing 3500 years before the birth of Christ. Speech then, is a recent development in the history of the world and its life.

Ontogenetic development of speech

Speech is acquired by the process of learning, which may be defined as the change in behaviour and perception of an organism as a consequence of its experience. A baby produces sound by crying as soon as it is born and, after a month, the cry becomes differentiated so that a mother appreciates its particular significance. As early as 2 months, an infant recognises the human voice, and soon after begins babbling: this is an essential part in the development of speech since it is a means of autostimulation (auditory feedback): the baby will stop babbling with any auditory stimulus—particularly if spoken to. At 6 months, the infant will distinguish between affectionate and scolding terms, and about this time the babbling is rhythmic and becomes lalling. At about 9 months of age, the child recognises familiar words and says 'Mama' and 'Dada'. It repeats words it hears—echolalia or psittacism, ('psittakos'—a parrot). The child loses nearly all the babbling sounds when it begins to articulate, and these sounds may be repeated for some time, e.g. 'a', 'l' and 'r'. Some children pass through a mute period between the babbling and language learning periods. In all languages, vowels are learned before consonants, the first vowel learned is an 'a', and the first consonant is an 'm'.

At 12 months of age, there will be a response to simple commands, and by 18 months the infant will acquire several words, many of which are peculiar to the child (idioglossia) but about 10–20 of these are meaningful. Although the learning of speech is relatively slow in the first 18 months, it is rapid for the next year, so that by the age of 2½ years the child can say two-word phrases. The rate of learning slows off at the age of 2½ years, the child acquiring about 500 new words each year and fully acquired speech—involving the use of sentences—comes gradually during the next few years.

The rapidity of learning depends not only on intelligence, but on the stimulation to speak, e.g. the home atmosphere and the social class of the parents. An only child is more likely to develop speech earlier than twins; the child of bilingual parents and a child in an orphanage are often slower than average.

The laborious learning of words, movements and reactions during early childhood depends on a system of repetitions and copying, trial and error. When the infant learns his first word, he has been listening to sounds of both himself and his mother; both use their personal pleasure as a facilitating mechanism, so that the sound is repeated in order to experience the pleasure again. When a child says 'Dada' he is repeating what he hears and then he correlates this with the seeing of a man; this necessitates remembering what the man looks like, and experiencing a feeling of familiarity and pleasure at the sight. The first process of repeating sounds soon becomes associated with the receptive systems, especially vision. The various sensations, including those from the muscles of the mouth and larynx, are essential for the registration of the neuronal patterns required to make the various noises that result in speech. The subsequent development of vocabulary and grammar is an elaboration of the more fundamental mechanism of registration. Learning to read and write, and correct spelling, involves many complex processes as does the capacity to name an object. Writing and reading are then learnt according to a programme and this capacity for learning is developed so that further knowledge can be superimposed. The neurological mechanisms depend partly on the repetition of previous responses; this is closely concerned with memory, which in its simplest form is the ability to repeat or recall a previous stimulus.

Animals learn to respond to sights, sounds and other sensations with motor reactions which may include making a noise; man has learned to produce a great variety of noises in relation to different objects, activities and feelings; in doing this, he uses highly specialised parts of his brain. Language and speech, as well as the related faculties of memory, learning and calculation are dependent on brain mechanisms which are integrated in, and controlled by, the cerebral hemispheres.

CHAPTER 2

THE BRAIN AND ITS FUNCTIONS

The brain is the most complicated organ of the body. It is composed of a complex network of nerve cells and fibres, requiring a rich blood supply (see Chapter 12) so that adequate oxygen, glucose, vitamins etc. are made available for metabolism. Restriction of these requirements will impair brain function and destruction of the nerve cells will lead to irreversible disorders.

Embryologically the anterior end of the central nervous system is modified into three parts, viz. the fore-brain, mid-brain and hind-brain. With development these parts increase in size and complexity, so that an adult human brain consists of many folded areas (gyri) with fissures in between (sulci). This convolutional pattern enables man to have the maximum amount of cerebral cortex in the smallest possible volume.

The surface of the brain (cortex) comprises the grey matter, which contains the nerve *cells* (neurones) and covers the underlying white matter which consists mainly of nerve *fibres*. There are also aggregations of neurones (nuclei) forming the basal ganglia which lie in the depths of each cerebral hemisphere. The cerebral hemispheres are joined together by the corpus callosum and each is connected with the brain stem by the cerebral peduncles. The brain stem has three parts; mid-brain, pons and medulla (or bulb).

The cerebellum consists of right and left cerebellar hemispheres, joined in the mid line by the vermis. Each cerebellar hemisphere is connected to the corresponding side of the brain stem by three cerebellar peduncles; superior (brachium conjunctivum), middle (brachium pontis) and inferior (restiform body).

Each cerebral hemisphere consists of frontal, parietal, temporal and occipital lobes (see Fig. 1). The central (Rolandic) fissure separates the frontal from the parietal lobe. The lateral (Sylvian) fissure demarcates the upper part of the temporal lobe. The

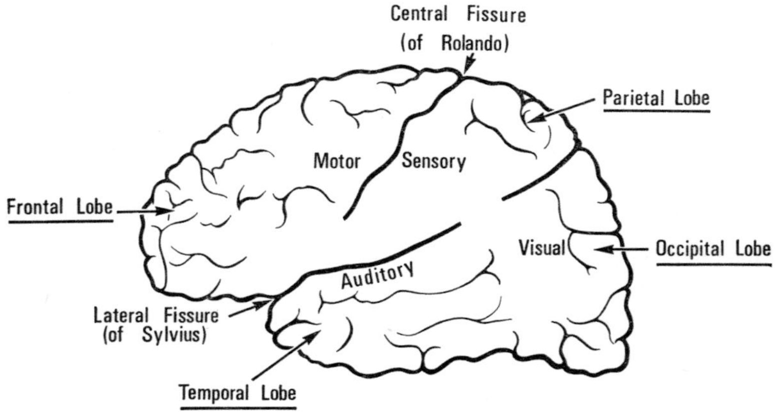

FIG. 1. Diagram of the lateral surface of the left cerebral hemisphere.

occipital lobe is the posterior part of the hemisphere, containing the calcarine (visual) cortex. Many of the main gyri are named and the whole cortex has been divided into anatomical regions, numbered as Brodmann's areas.

The phrenologists considered that the fissures divided the brain into regions which were concerned with personality characteristics, for example, intelligence, memory and piety. These attempts to localise specific function to certain anatomical areas conflicted with the view that the brain was an amorphous organ whose cells, like the cells of the liver, could function in many capacities. Localisation of speech function within the brain was suggested by Broca in 1861, and subsequent observations including experiments using electrical stimulation have shown that other important functions are controlled by specific parts of the brain. Thus the cerebral control of movements is located in the precentral gyrus which is the main motor area. The postcentral gyrus represents sensory functions; the visual cortex is in the occipital lobe. There are also so-called non-committed areas of the brain, for example in the frontal lobes, containing association fibres so that the brain can function as a whole.

THE SPEECH AREA

The surface markings of the area of the dominant cerebral hemisphere controlling speech and language functions are shown in Fig. 2. This includes the lowermost part of the pre-central gyrus (Broca's area) and post-central gyrus, the supramarginal and angular gyri, the inferior parietal gyri and upper part of the temporal lobe (Wernicke's area). The disorders of speech due to lesions in this area are described in Chapter 5. The concept of *cerebral dominance* is discussed in Chapter 4.

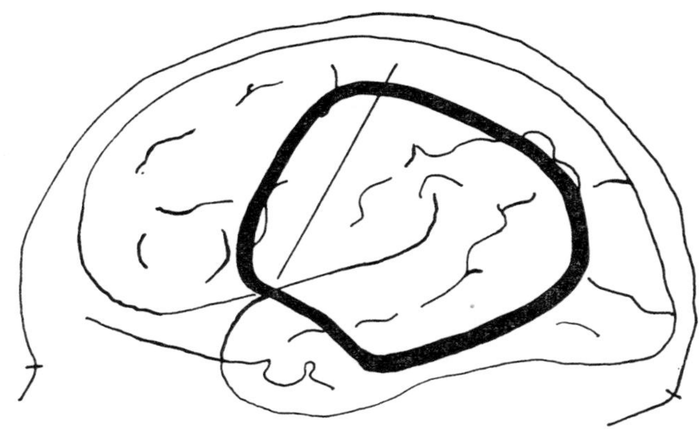

FIG. 2. The thick line indicates the limits of the area of the brain within which a small wound will cause aphasia (Russell W. R. 1963). The speech area thus lies within this and includes Broca's and Wernicke's areas. (Reproduced by permission of the author and the *Lancet*).

THE FRONTAL LOBES

The pre-central gyrus in each cerebral hemisphere contains the motor cortex, in which the large motor nerve cells (Betz cells) are situated. The face is represented by the lower-most part in the inferior frontal region, there is a large area for the hand and upper limb in the middle, and the leg area is uppermost (viz. in the parasagittal region) and extends over the medial surface of the hemisphere. The area anterior to the pre-central gyrus is called the pre-motor cortex, which covers a large association area for co-ordination of motor function.

part of everyday life and social necessity. The primitive instincts of a child normally become inhibited by conditioning and, with maturity, customs and etiquette are learnt so that impulses, emotions and actions are suppressed to conform with the requirements of the environment.

Voluntary control of movements of the head and neck and eye movements are also associated with frontal lobe function, as is control of the bladder and sexual functions.

Frontal Lobe Syndromes

Patients with frontal lobe disorders manifest disinhibition, with inadequately controlled, aggressive or anti-social behaviour, as well as dementia (see Chapter 9), deterioration of personality and intellect, slowness of thought and loss of initiative. The mental changes resulting from frontal lobe lesions include defects of emotional control; there is a tendency to laugh childishly or inappropriately, with inability to realise the true seriousness of situations, for example, lack of insight into the gravity of medical disability. Changes in mood range from the feeling of well-being or excessive cheerfulness (euphoria) which is inappropriate and pathological, to mania; alternatively the patient becomes depressed, miserable and melancholic without adequate reason.

Lesions in the motor area will cause weakness in the opposite side of the body, i.e. the face, arm or leg, according to the situation and extent of the lesion. The terms *hemiparesis* or *hemiplegia* are used to describe respectively weakness or paralysis of one half of the body, (i.e. face, arm and leg); *monoplegia* means paralysis of one limb, either arm or leg (see Chapter 6).

THE PARIETAL LOBES

The parietal lobes are the main receiving areas for sensory impulses and stimuli. Parts of the body are represented in the contralateral sensory cortex of the post-central gyrus in the same way as on the motor side. The sensory impulses travel from the end organs in the skin, muscles, joints and other tissues of the body and are conveyed proximally in centripetal fashion via the sensory (spinal and cranial) nerves. From the dorsal root ganglia, the fibres of the posterior nerve roots enter the spinal cord and form the main sensory tracts, which pass up via the brain stem to the first receiving station in the thalamus. The impulses are then relayed from the thalamus through the posterior part of the internal capsule and radiate out to the appropriate parts of the sensory cortex.

Basic sensations such as touch pass to the post-central gyrus, whereas impulses for finer discrimination and interpretation pass to the larger area of the parietal lobe posterior to the post-central gyrus. These finer discriminative functions are concerned with size, shape and consistency of substances which are felt and allow differentiation of complicated sensations, appreciation of the sense of position of the opposite side of the body, and the location of particular parts of the body in space. This is a highly developed function which becomes automatic, so that the position and movement of a hand is known both in relation to a given object and also in relation to other parts of the body. The orientation in space and appreciation of the body-image (see page 20) is dependent upon the function of the association areas of the parietal region. It is linked with the visual cortex in the occipital region and performance of many manoeuvres is improved by seeing.

Parietal Lobe Syndromes

Damage to the sensory pathways or receiving areas in one parietal lobe will cause a contralateral hemianaesthesia, i.e. impairment of sensation on the opposite side of the body. If the lesion is localised, the sensory loss may be limited—e.g. to the hand or leg. Parietal lobe lesions may also cause various types of apraxia and agnosia, disorientation and disturbances of the body image (see Chapter 3) and a homonymous hemianopia if the optic radiation is involved (see page 15).

THE TEMPORAL LOBES

A large part of the temporal lobe of the dominant cerebral hemisphere is concerned with speech, particularly the middle zone of the upper temporal convolution (Wernicke's area). This forms part of the main auditory-receptive centre for the assimilation and interpretation of sounds required for the understanding of speech. The medial part of each temporal lobe includes the uncus, hippocampus and amygdaloid body which are concerned with *memory* and the *sense of smell.* The hippocampus is linked with the mamillary bodies (corpora mamillaria) via the fornix of the corpus callosum, which also forms a connection with the hippocampus of the opposite temporal lobe.

Memory

Memory depends on the capacity of the C.N.S. to perform actions repeatedly and establish store houses of neuronal patterns. The use of the word 'memory' is sometimes restricted to the higher psychological aspects of recalling stored material, which is used with ever-increasing confidence as the individual matures. Unfortunately the physiological mechanisms underlying the simplest memory, such as remembering how to walk, are little understood, but it is thought that the key structures controlling memory are the synapses (see page 36) rather than the neurones themselves. The urge to remember depends greatly on the stimulus of interest, attention and the emotions, joy, fear, love, hate, etc. The fronto-hypothalamic system is responsible for some of this emotional drive, but it is the fronto-temporal neuronal system, particularly in the dominant hemisphere, which facilitates the highly elaborate activity required for speech, memory, thought, initiative and the general control of behaviour. The cortical connections with the thalamus and the opposite cerebral hemisphere are also important so that severe disorganisation may also result from lesions of the deeper structures.

Recently acquired memories are formed from information reaching the sensory-receiving areas including the visual and auditory cortex, and evidence suggests that the hippocampus, fornix of the corpus callosum and mamillary bodies form a facilitating mechanism for the storage of current events and learning new material. *Old established memories* on the other hand appear to depend on a different mechanism, maintained by the spontaneous activity of neurones, which is less vulnerable to degenerative and disease processes. Thus the activity of the hippocampal system which facilitates the storage of current events tends to decline in old age, and this accounts for the forgetfulness of old people who fail to remember day to day happenings yet refer repeatedly to events of the past.

Amnesia (loss of memory) mainly for recent events and confusion of thought are features of concussion following a head injury.

Small wounds of the dominant left temporal lobe have a longer period of post-traumatic amnesia when compared with those of the right temporal lobe and other parts of the brain. Memory is regained when hippocampal function recovers or if the hippocampus of the opposite hemisphere takes over. After bilateral excision of the temporal lobes, there is a striking loss of ability to store current events, while remote memories are conserved. A similar effect is seen in patients with Korsakoff's psychosis (due to vitamin B_1 deficiency, e.g. resulting from alcoholism) in which there are lesions in the corpora mamillaria.

Knowledge and capacity for thought are closely linked with memory for names, words, languages and music, which are probably stored in the cortex and association areas of the temporal lobe, whereas memory for the motor and sensory skills seems to be a function of the frontal and parietal lobes. All these may be disorganised in lesions causing aphasia, which may also interfere with the activity of the system whereby memories are preserved. Thought is of little avail without the retention of knowledge, and both recently acquired and long established memories are important for every facet of the speech mechanism, whether it be of a sound, a sight, the capacity to make a remembered noise in speaking, or movement in writing. Thus the formulation of thoughts and their transfer into words, as well as the ability to learn and judge, have to be integrated with memories derived from things that have been heard and seen.

Many people depend greatly on visual memory, and the use of the storage systems is also required when reading. This process includes recognition of the visual patterns of the letters and words and of the associations which add a 'meaning' to the words (though we have little knowledge of what meaning involves in physiological terms). Reading also demands the capacity to remember what is read for long enough to correlate it with later pages. The inability to remember what has been read might be due to a lesion either of the hippocampus or of the storage mechanisms in the posterior parietal lobes.

In temporal lobe epilepsy (see Chapter 10) memories and feelings of familiarity (déjà-vu sensations) are provoked in attacks, and the various hallucinations which occur can be regarded as forced or distorted memories. These features of temporal lobe attacks mimic or reflect the normal facilitating mechanisms, the epileptic activity stimulating the storage systems concerned with the special senses in the hippocampus.

Lesions confined to the temporal lobe cause no motor or sensory changes on the opposite side of the body but may involve the optic radiation and produce contralateral homonymous visual field defects (see page 15). The anterior 5–6 cm. of one temporal lobe can be removed surgically (temporal lobectomy) without any obvious clinical sequelae.

THE OCCIPITAL LOBES

These contain the calcarine (visual) cortex. A complete lesion on one side will give a homonymous hemianopia on the opposite side (see Fig. 4 (c)). Partial lesions of one occipital lobe will cause congruous defects or scotomata in the homonymous visual fields of various shapes, according to the exact extent of the lesion.

THE OPTIC RADIATION

The fibres forming this part of the visual pathway lie deep in the temporal and parietal lobes and convey impulses from the lateral geniculate body on each side to the visual cortex in the occipital lobe. A lesion of the temporal lobe may initially involve the lower part of the optic radiation as it passes round the temporal horn of the lateral ventricle and so cause contralateral homonymous *upper* quadrantic visual field defects (see Fig. 4 (a)). A lesion of the parietal lobe may involve the upper part of the optic radiation and so cause contralateral homonymous *lower* quadrantic visual field defects (see Fig. 4 (b)). If either temporal or parietal lobe lesions extend to involve the whole of the optic radiation, then a complete contralateral homonymous hemianopia will result (see Fig. 4 (c)).

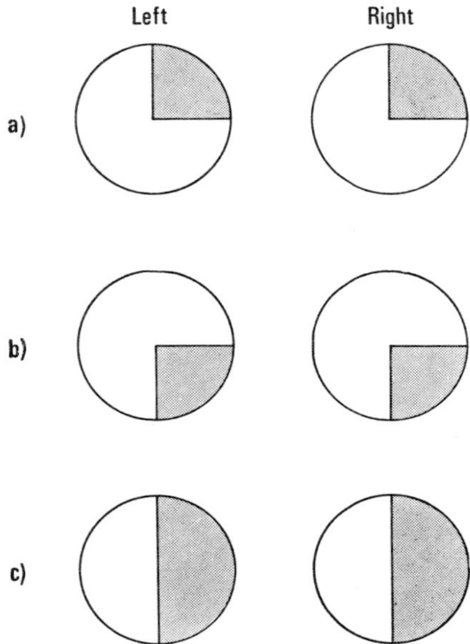

FIG. 4. Visual field defects (represented by shaded areas):
(a) right homonymous upper quadrantic.
(b) right homonymous lower quadrantic.
(c) right homonymous hemianopia.

CHAPTER 3

APRAXIA AND AGNOSIA

APRAXIA

The ability to perform purposeful movements and complicated skills is gradually learned by practice and experience; these motor activities are organised and stored by the association areas of the frontal and parietal lobes. Apraxia is the loss of skill required for complex actions due to inability to perform specific movements at will, yet the same movements can be performed in isolation or involuntarily. There is no paralysis and the individual muscles can participate in other movements. The causative lesion involves the relevant association areas representing movements rather than individual muscles, and interferes with the control of movements by the corresponding part of the motor cortex, although the fibres forming the main motor pathway remain intact.

In general, the more recently acquired actions are lost first, so that in mild cases the less complicated and primitive skills are preserved. In severe forms the patient regresses to a state comparable to infancy with inco-ordinate movements affecting actions such as walking or standing. These movements, automatic in adult life, are based on the concept of 'kinetic engrams' and the disturbances of these have been called limb-kinetic, innervatory or cortical apraxia.

Ideomotor apraxia is the term suggested when the kinetic engrams are present, the patient has no difficulty in formulating the idea of the act which he wishes to carry out but finds himself unable to execute it. Simple tests such as asking a patient to salute, make a fist or shake hands, reveal an ideomotor apraxia whereas other movements such as grasping an object can be done automatically.

Ideational apraxia is when the conception of the movement is faulty, for example, on being asked to light a cigarette, the patient puts the match into his mouth instead of the cigarette. This type is closely linked with ideomotor apraxia and agnosia as there is clearly a failure to recognise the nature or use of the object for which the movements are required. In severe forms, ideational apraxia is combined with ideomotor apraxia.

There may also be an inability to dress or undress (*dressing apraxia*), construct models from blocks or letters with matches (*constructional apraxia*).

With regard to speech, apraxia of the lips or tongue is relatively common and will produce an apraxic dysarthria, automatic movements of the tongue and facial muscles being preserved. Facial apraxia is not uncommonly associated with expressive and nominal aphasia. Constructional apraxia may interfere with drawing or writing, and is thus a cause of dysgraphia which should be distinguished from that resulting from a specific defect of language.

Although apraxia is manifest as a motor disability, there is often an element of agnosia as well; in dressing apraxia, the patient may be unable to relate the spatial forms of his garments to that of his body, and in constructional apraxia the patient may be unaware of the inadequacy of his achievement and so there may be defective recognition both of the model and the copy.

The site of the lesion causing apraxia is usually the post-central area of the parietal lobe but the temporal lobe is sometimes involved. Lesions causing ideational and ideomotor apraxia are usually bilateral but constructional apraxia may be caused by a lesion in either hemisphere, and dressing apraxia by a lesion of the non-dominant hemisphere.

AGNOSIA

The ability to interpret sensory stimuli which are conveyed to the brain from the special senses (e.g. visual and auditory) and from other parts of the body (e.g. touch) is a function of the cerebral hemispheres. The cortex of the temporal, parietal and occipital lobes are mainly concerned with the processes of recognition or perception of sensory stimuli (gnosis). This implies that the crude sensory stimuli acquire significance by collation with previous experiences stored as memories in the appropriate association areas.

Agnosia, a term first introduced by Freud in 1891, means a loss of this ability to recognise these sensory experiences; it is a defect of perception due to a disorder of cerebral mechanisms. The lesions causing the defects involve localised areas of the cerebral cortex and their association areas, the primary sensory pathways being intact. The various types of agnosia depend on the sensory modality involved.

Visual Agnosia

Visual agnosia was called 'imperception' by Hughlings Jackson and various types are now described.

Visual object agnosia is the inability to recognise objects seen, this failure not being attributable to defects of vision or to general intellectual impairment. Not only is there failure to recognise an object but also what the object is used for, (ct: nominal aphasia, in which the object cannot be named but its nature or use can often be described). A patient with visual agnosia is usually able to name the object if allowed to feel it. The lesion responsible for visual object agnosia is thought to be in the cortex of the 2nd and 3rd occipital convolutions or possibly in the splenium of the corpus callosum, through which pass fibres linking the visual cortex of the two hemispheres.

Visual object agnosia is sometimes associated with tactile agnosia, alexia, constructional apraxia and Gerstmann's syndrome (see page 20).

Dyslexia (see Chapters 5 and 16) may also be a type of visual agnosia, when the patterns produced by letters, words, numbers or music fail to be recognised or understood. The meaning must be stored in order to obtain the sequence of what follows. A homonymous hemianopia due to lesions of the optic radiation may also cause difficulty with reading; but the difficulties due to defects of visual acuity and of the visual fields differ from dyslexia which concerns the problems of using and understanding visual symbol patterns. The visual pathways of the brain play a large part in language, learning, memory and thought; congenitally blind patients develop speech mechanisms differently (Critchley, 1953).

Spelling difficulties may also be due to disturbances of visual imagery due to lesions in the posterior parietal region.

Many other types of visual agnosia have been described. *Prosopagnosia* is a name given to the failure to recognise faces, normally well-known. *Simultanagnosia* is the failure to appreciate the meaning of a complex picture or recognise a combination of details although the individual elements and details are correctly recognised. This is also called visual extinction and indicates a lesion of the posterior temporal or parietal lobe. Visual inattention is the failure to see an object on one side when shown objects on both sides of the visual field simultaneously, there being no defect when each object is shown separately. *Agnosia for colours* has to be distinguished from nominal aphasia in which the colours are recognised but cannot be named. *Visual disorientation* may include defective visual localisation, loss of visual imagery, loss of stereoscopic vision and spatial agnosia. *Loss of topographical memory* may also occur independently of other forms of visual disorientation and of loss of memory for objects.

Auditory Agnosia

In auditory agnosia, hearing is not impaired but there is an inability to recognise or distinguish the sounds which are heard due to a lesion of the left superior temporal convolution. With the eyes closed or covered, the patient cannot recognise familiar noises, such as the jingling of keys or coins. The loss of recognition of musical sounds is called *sensory amusia.* Failure to understand spoken speech (word deafness or receptive aphasia) may also be a form of auditory agnosia.

Tactile Agnosia

Tactile agnosia, the failure to recognise objects by touch, is also called *astereognosis*. Sensation in the hands is otherwise normal, but the patient fails to recognise the shape, size or consistency of the object, which is placed in his hand without his being allowed to see it. Tactile agnosia may occur without visual agnosia, so that patients can then recognise by sight what they cannot recognise by feel. The lesion responsible is thought to be in the supramarginal gyrus of the parietal lobe, and there is evidence that in right handed persons bilateral tactile agnosia may be produced by a lesion in this area of the left cerebral hemisphere, suggesting that there may be dominance for tactile recognition.

The body image

Movements of all parts of our body both in relation to each other and to the external environment, as well as perception and recognition, are integrated so that we develop a body schema or awareness of our body image. Learning and memory mechanisms allow the use of previous experiences so that mental and physical performances become automatic or can be geared to changes in oneself or in the environment. This concept of the body image implies that a storage, collating and selecting system exists in the association areas, particularly of the parietal lobes.

Somatagnosia is the name given to disorders of the body schema; these include imperception or neglect of parts of the body (*autotopagnosia*) right-left disorientation (i.e. the inability to distinguish right from left) and denial of disability, e.g. unawareness of a hemiplegic limb (*anosognosia*). Another example is seen in some patients with complete cortical blindness who deny that they are blind but confabulate that they can see (*Anton's syndrome*).

The variety of possible defects, single and combined, is considerable. One such combination is *Gerstmann's syndrome*, viz: finger agnosia (an inability of the patient to recognise or identify his own fingers or those of the observer) right-left disorientation, agraphia and acalculia.

Site of lesions causing agnosia

Gerstmann's syndrome results from a lesion of the left supramarginal and angular gyri, but there is controversy as to whether this is a distinct entity or merely represents one of a variety of combined defects resulting from lesions of the parietal cortex. Unilateral spatial agnosia and prosopagnosia are usually due to a parieto-occipital lesion of the non-dominant hemisphere. In other types of agnosia the lesions are usually extensive and may be bilateral but it would be wrong to suggest that there is an exact anatomical localisation for each type of agnosia.

CHAPTER 4

CEREBRAL DOMINANCE

The cerebral hemisphere controlling speech is the dominant hemisphere, and the concept of cerebral dominance is closely related to the problems of aphasia. Bouillard in 1865 suggested that cerebral dominance for speech and handedness were in some way interconnected and later Hughlings Jackson introduced his concept of the 'leading hemisphere', implying a physiological rather than any anatomical difference between the two hemispheres. However recent studies have shown that the dominant parietal lobe controlling speech, spatial orientation and praxis is slightly larger and contains more nerve cells than the non-dominant parietal lobe. Furthermore the electroencephalogram often shows a lower voltage alpha rhythm over the dominant hemisphere.

Laterality implies that one side is preferred when performing certain skills, for example with the hand, foot or eye. Usually there is consistence in the side preferred for a particular skill but laterality depends upon the skill tested, e.g. a person may write with the left hand and throw a ball with the right, yet prefer to kick a ball with the left foot; this is called mixed laterality or mixed dominance. Although there may be a preferred eye, e.g. in looking through a telescope or kaleidoscope, this cannot be directly related to cerebral dominance since the nerve fibres from each eye go to both hemispheres. To test visual dominance, the choice of left or right visual fields would have to be tested. The relationship between eyedness and cerebral dominance may also depend upon which hand is preferred for holding the telescope.

Right handedness is a feature of the majority of people in all nations and such evidence as is available, e.g. from prehistoric cave paintings, suggests that this has always been so. It is not known for certain whether dextrality is an organic or cultural heritage—even the accepted familial trend of sinistrality is unhelpful since this could be either genetic or environmental (or both).

An infant does not show any preference for either hand until the age of about 9 months when speech begins. Handedness slowly becomes established—with speech—after the age of two, and laterality is undoubtedly governed in some cases by agenesis or damage of one cerebral hemisphere. It is now generally recognised that there are varying degrees of laterality, some people being more strongly right handed than others. True ambidexterity, i.e. the ability to use either hand equally well, is probably quite rare.

It used to be thought that the left cerebral hemisphere was dominant for speech in right handers and the right hemisphere in left handers. However in 1959 Penfield and Roberts concluded from studies of cortical stimulation and excision in patients with epilepsy that the left cerebral hemisphere was dominant for speech in nearly everyone, whether left handed or right handed, provided that one excluded cases of pathological left handedness, i.e. due to trauma or disease of the left hemisphere at birth or during infancy. The present position regarding the relationship between cerebral dominance and handedness is that the left cerebral hemisphere is almost always dominant for speech in right handers with very rare exceptions. The left cerebral hemisphere is also dominant for speech in a proportion (probably 50%) of left handers. There are other left handers whose right cerebral hemisphere is dominant and in these cases there is by no means always evidence of trauma or disease to the left hemisphere at birth or during infancy. Confirmation of this view has been obtained from the study of brain wounds (Russell and Espir, 1961) and cases of post-traumatic epilepsy having an aphasic aura (see Chapter 10) and more recently from the technique of intracarotid arterial injection (Milner, Branch and Rasmussen, 1964). It is also possible that in some cases both hemispheres may contribute to language functions without definite dominance on one side; this is the concept of *cerebral ambilaterality* suggested by Zangwill (1960).

Left handedness

Left handed subjects are those who prefer to use the left hand for the performance of the majority of one handed motor skills, e.g. throwing a ball and using a racket; this may include preference for kicking a ball with the left foot. The incidence of left handedness in the general population ranges from 5–10%. It may be thought that left handers who write with the left hand are more strongly left handed than left handers who write with the right hand and that they would be more likely to have the right hemisphere dominant or perhaps have cerebral ambilaterality; but whether a left hander uses his left or right hand for writing does not necessarily indicate which hemisphere is dominant. Thus some left handers who write with the left hand are rendered aphasic from left hemisphere lesions, and others, also left handed writers, are rendered aphasic from right hemisphere lesions; the same applies to left handers who write with the right hand.

Individual variation in the degree of laterality is common amongst left handers, and many use their right hand more often and more skilfully than right handers use their left.

CHAPTER 5

DYSPHASIA

History

Probably the earliest case of aphasia ever recorded is in the first chapter of the Gospel according to St. Luke, where Zacharias was struck dumb but could still write (v.v. 20–22, & 62–64), and the next in Roman times, when about A.D. 30 Valerius Maximus described a learned man of Athens who lost his memory for letters after being struck by a stone. There were several reports of aphasia in the seventeenth and eighteenth centuries by Linnaeus the great botanist, Morgagni, Heberden and also Goethe in his novel 'Wilhelm Meister'.

The early descriptions explained aphasia on a motor basis in terms of paralysis of the tongue and other organs of speech ('The dead palsy'), and occasionally as part of a general loss of mental faculties (Willis, 1683). A century later, when it was observed that aphasia could occur without motor paralysis and without overall dementia, the phenomenon was classed as a defect of memory. With the influence of phrenological studies in the nineteenth century, specific cerebral lesions of the organ of language were described.

In April 1861 Dr. Paul Broca had under his care at the Bicêtre Hospital in Paris a speechless hemiplegic patient. The patient eventually died and, at post mortem examination, a cavity the size of a hen's egg was found in the posterior third of the left second and third frontal convolutions (the equivalent of Brodmann's area 44). This was demonstrated by Broca at a meeting of the Société d'Anthropologie de Paris and as similar cases were collected, he formed the axiom—'on parle avec l'hémisphère gauche'. (There is controversy as to whether the priority given to Broca for his discovery is justified. Dr. Mark Dax of Montpellier, according to his son Gustave, had written a paper in 1836 to the effect that lesions interfering with speech lay in the left hemisphere. This paper was not published until 1865 and Broca did not know about it at the time of his original communication). Broca called the speech disorder 'aphemia'; previously it had been called 'alalia'. The term aphasia, which had been used in a philosophical sense in the second century A.D. by the Romans, was reintroduced by Trousseau in 1864. Following this, the concept of cerebral dominance was developed.

During the last 100 years, there has been considerable debate as to the best way in which to classify the disorders of speech which results from a lesion in the dominant hemisphere, and writers on the subject have included Hughlings Jackson in this country, Charcot, Marie and Dejerine in France, and Henschen and Kleist in Germany.

As mentioned in Chapter 2, there is still controversy as to whether various parts of the cortex are solely concerned with specific functions and whether a lesion of part of the speech mechanism will produce some impairment of all other aspects. Pierre Marie in 1906 attacked all the existing theories regarding aphasia (and for this reason was described by Head as 'the Iconoclast') and later in 1917, with his colleague Foix, demonstrated the anatomical extent of the speech territory from a study of brain wounds identifying five zones, lesions of which produced particular varieties of speech disorders. They concluded that pure motor aphasia ('anarthrie') was the only speech disorder that could occur in isolation. In 1926 Head reported a series of 26 cases and his work achieved great significance from the fine detail in which his patients were studied and the brilliant discussion of the problems revealed by the clinical findings. Kleist (1934) reported detailed studies of similar material from Germany but, unlike Head, he attempted to elucidate a large number of clinical syndromes, each corresponding with small areas of cortical damage. Henschen (1920, 1922) also attempted to localise separate aspects of language function with evidence from over 1300 cases in the literature.

Whereas before and during the early part of the twentietn century, most workers concentrated on localisation of speech functions and tended to ignore their setting in the hierarchy of higher cerebral function, the pendulum has swung back again to the holistic approach linking speech with memory and the other mental faculties.

The patho-physiology of aphasia is the most difficult in neurology. A word may be regarded as a sequence of auditory events (phonemes) and there is an average of 5 phonemes per word. English is normally spoken at the rate of 120 words per minute, so each phoneme lasts about 10 milliseconds (1/100th. sec). Some phonemes have more significance than others and consonants provide more information than vowels (so that some languages, e.g. Hebrew, can dispense with the latter). Not every phoneme is appreciated but there is a redundancy in speech so that other factors, such as rhythm and intonation, are important.

Definition

Dysphasia may be defined as the loss of ability to formulate, express or understand the meaning of spoken words; in addition, there may be failure to understand written words (dyslexia), gestures, signs (asymbolia) or music (amusia). With dysphasia there is confusion in the expression and understanding of speech and language due to a focal cerebral lesion; it has to be distinguished from general mental confusion which results from more diffuse disorders of cerebral function. This distinction is often difficult but mental confusion includes disturbances of thought processes, intellectual ability and behaviour as well as speech and memory.

The terms aphasia (alexia etc) strictly indicate a complete loss of function, whereas dysphasia (dyslexia etc) imply partial loss; however the prefix a- and dys- are often used interchangeably.

Clinical Types

The main division is into expressive or executive defects (*motor dysphasia*) and receptive defects (*sensory dysphasia*). Although either expressive or receptive defects may predominate, elements of both are usually present. Speech requires the combined activity of the mechanisms of movement, hearing, and seeing and these are completely interdependent; a lesion, even a small one, that interrupts connections between them may cause catastrophic effects on all aspects of speech. This type has been called *central* or *global aphasia*.

Since speech is originally developed in relation to hearing words, auditory organisation remains the fundamental scaffolding on which all else is built. Thus damage to the auditory area and its storage systems puts most aspects of speech out of action. Speech is heard but not understood by the patient (*word deafness*) and if he talks it is unintelligible (*jargon*). Because of this patients are almost devoid of rational thought or action. Writing is usually impossible (*dysgraphia*) although the ability to copy letters may be preserved, and reading will also be lost (*dyslexia*). This global effect suggests that even if parts of the speech mechanisms are normal, they are rendered useless by damage to the central speech organisation.

Inability to name objects is called *nominal* or *amnestic* dysphasia. Patients may be unable to construct sentences (*syntactical dysphasia*) or use a jumble of meaningless words (*jargon dysphasia*). These are descriptive clinical divisions which may be associated with receptive or expressive defects. Patients with expressive dysphasia commonly realise their disability and, for this reason, are disinclined to attempt to speak. Those which receptive or sensory dysphasia commonly do not realise their mistakes and may talk excessively (*logorrhoea*). Disturbances of inflexion, stress and rhythm (*dysprosody*) are other features which may occur.

Expressive dysphasia is due to a lesion in the region of the inferior frontal convolution of the dominant cerebral hemisphere (Broca's area) or of its connections; sensory dysphasia to a lesion in the posterior temporal or temporo-parietal region of the dominant hemisphere (Wernicke's area) or of its connections.

Dysphasia, in addition to causing difficulty in speaking, often affects the intellect as well but the patient retains *non-intellectual speech*. This consists of:

(1) *Emotional utterances*—e.g. (a) ejaculations or expostulations.
 (b) 'Yes' and 'No' which are primitive words in the sense that they are among the first to be learnt.
 (c) other words used inappropriately or without regard to their proper sense.
 (d) *jargon*, where words are meaningless and unintelligible.
 (e) *recurrent utterances* of words or phrases which are sometimes those that were used just before lesion occurred.

(2) *automatic speech:* such as songs and poems.

(3) *serial speech:* such as the alphabet, days of the week or months of the year.

(4) *social gesture speech* such as 'How do you do' or 'Goodbye'.

Some of these forms of speech may be retained by virtue of the contribution by the non-dominant hemisphere.

Expressive Dysphasia

This is similar to the 'verbal aphasia' of Head, in which there is defective formation of words and when severe, the patient may be unable to say anything. In the less severe form, or during recovery, the patient may be able to speak in a telegram style leaving out prepositions and conjunctions (*telegrammatism*), with a general poverty of spontaneous speech. There may be grammatical errors (*paragrammatism* or *syntactical aphasia*) with confusion of articles and conjunctions. Disorders of word formation, resulting in faulty pronunciation (*cortical* or *apraxic dysarthria*) occur sometimes with reversion to spoonerisms, use of wrong words and difficulty with word finding. *Perseveration* of words is also a characteristic feature; it is the inappropriate repetition of the same reply to different questions. *Paraphasia* is the name given to disorders of sentence formation and is not to be confused with *periphrasis*, a circumlocutory way of saying things which also occurs in this type of dysphasia.

Some patients are unaware of their mistakes but those with nominal aphasia will usually recognise the correct name when it is offered. This could be due to a loss of memory for the appropriate word (amnestic aphasia). There may also be a failure to recognise the significance or intention of words or phrases (*semantic aphasia*).

Pure word dumbness is another type of expressive aphasia with loss of spontaneous speech and writing, and inability to read aloud although the patient is still able to repeat words or phrases and write by copying or on dictation. Such patients are able to tap out the number of syllables in a word (which patients with other types of expressive aphasia cannot do). A possible explanation is that there is an interruption between the cortical centre for storage of words and the motor pathways of articulation.

Receptive Aphasia

Auditory—word deafness

In auditory—word deafness, words although heard are not understood, and fail to convey their normal meaning. In a less severe form, individual words may be recognised and understood but the meaning of sentences is not appreciated. This could be classified as an agnosia for words and there may even be auditory agnosia for sounds so that a patient may be unable to interpret the significance of sounds, for example, the rattle of a bunch of keys.

These types of 'deafness' are not due to any defect of the peripheral mechanism of hearing, but there is a failure to appreciate the significance or meaning of sounds transmitted to, or received by, the auditory area. If this part of the dominant hemisphere is damaged, receptive dysphasia and, when severe, auditory agnosia are likely to result. If damage is confined to the corresponding part of the non-dominant hemisphere, there is no noticeable effect. Destruction of the auditory areas bilaterally causes cortical deafness, i.e. a complete failure to recognise any sound even though the peripheral mechanism for hearing is intact. Thus the non-dominant hemisphere contributes to the control of speech by the dominant hemisphere, the corpus callosum being the main connection between the two hemispheres. Recovery of speech after severe lesions of the dominant left hemisphere may also depend on the functioning of the right hemisphere, and an additional lesion of the *right* parietal lobe or corpus callosum will probably prevent the redevelopment of language functions.

THE EXAMINATION OF THE APHASIC PATIENT

There are many different methods of clinical and psychological assessment of aphasia, (e.g. Schuell's), and most differ only in detail and the order of tests performed.

It is important to remember that a dysphasic patient fatigues more easily than a normal person and that concentration is impaired; for these reasons several interviewing periods may be necessary. For clinical purposes the following routine proves helpful.

(1) Preliminary assessment of:
- (a) general mental state, e.g. disorientation in space and time, confusion.
- (b) hearing.

(c) vision, e.g. homonymous hemianopia or other visual field defect.
(d) motor function, e.g. hemiparesis.

(2) Cerebral dominance: which hand, leg or eye is preferred.

(3) Receptive function:
(a) response to spoken questions and commands, initially simple and then more complex.
If incorrect response note whether mistakes are recognised.
(b) response to written questions and commands, picking out from a group of objects the one that is written down.

(4) Expressive function:
(a) speech—spontaneity, quantity and fluency.
The correctness of word formation, sentence construction and reading.
The presence of emotional speech, the lack of propositional speech.
Singing better than speech.
Repetition of words and sentences.
Serial speech, e.g. letters of the alphabet, days of the week, months of the year, well known sayings.
In polyglot patients ascertain which languages have been lost.
Naming objects if nominal defect; can use of objects be described.
Recognition of correct names and colours.
(b) writing—spontaneous (not only name and address, which are often 'automatic') names of objects shown, writing to dictation, copy writing.
(c) spelling.

(5) Other symbolic functions:
reading numbers aloud.
Writing numbers to dictation.
Copying numbers, or copying numbers written as digits and numbers as words.
Copying geometric figures.
Drawing.
Calculation.
Music.

(6) Apraxia:
use of objects—e.g. matches, comb, scissors, eating utensils.

Simple movements—e.g. putting out tongue, showing teeth, waving goodbye, dressing.
Complicated actions.

(7) Agnosia and disorders of body image:
distinction between right and left, getting in and out of bed, finding way, recognition of objects, finger agnosia.

CAUSES OF APHASIA

The pathological conditions which most commonly cause aphasia are:

(1) Cerebral vascular disorders (see Chapter 12).
(2) Intracranial tumours (see Chapter 11).
(3) Cerebral abscess (see Chapter 13).
(4) Brain injuries.

In fact there are many diseases which can interfere with the cerebral control of speech and language. Aphasia is thus not a pathological diagnosis, but merely a manifestation of any lesion of the speech area. Occasionally it occurs as an isolated deficit, although in most cases there are associated disturbances of cerebral function, such as a right upper motor neurone type of facial weakness or hemiparesis. However the aphasia and hemiparesis may develop or recover independently of each other.

Aphasia may also occur as a transitory phenomenon in migraine or as the aura of a focal epileptic attack.

Developmental speech and language disorders are described separately in Chapter 16.

PROGNOSIS OF APHASIA

The degree of recovery from aphasia depends upon many factors, the chief being the following:

1. The site and extent of the lesion; e.g. which part and how much of the speech area has been affected, whether the non-dominant hemisphere and commissures have been damaged.

2. The cause of the lesion: e.g. whether the pathological process is reversible or progressive, benign or malignant.
3. Treatment of the cause: response to drugs or radiotherapy, whether surgical removal of a tumour has been total or partial.
4. Speech therapy: stage when started.
5. The severity and clinical type of dysphasia; the more severe the dysphasia, the greater the amount of recovery required. Severe receptive defects may make it impossible for speech therapy to be given. Associated language defects are also important e.g. dyslexia and dysgraphia.
6. (a) Associated non-language defects; e.g. impairment of other mental functions, particularly memory, apraxia and agnosia.

   (b) Other disabilities; e.g. defects of visual fields (homonymous hemianopia), ocular movements (diplopia), motor functions (hemiplegia), sensory functions (hemianaesthesia), epilepsy, dizziness.
7. (a) Psychological factors: e.g. inability to concentrate, to co-operate and to adjust to limitations, depression, emotional lability.

   (b) Environmental factors; e.g. home and social conditions, help from relatives, encouragement and reassurance.
8. Age: the older the patient, the poorer the prognosis.
9. Cerebral dominance: (see Chapter 4).
10. Premorbid language and intellectual ability, personality and temperament.

CHAPTER 6

DYSARTHRIA I

Dysarthria literally means disordered articulation and therefore could be due to local non-neurological causes such as cleft palate and loose fitting dentures. The term is perhaps better restricted to faulty pronunciation due to neuromuscular disorders.

The correct pronunciation of words (articulation) is dependent upon complex processes which control and co-ordinate the neuro-muscular system. The sounds recognised as words are produced by the vibration of the vocal cords in the larynx, caused by an outflow of air coming from the lungs; any interference with this mechanism produces weakness or hoarseness of the voice (dysphonia). The sounds are then given their correct form by movements of lips, tongue and palate and any abnormality of this system produces defects or difficulty in articulation, hypo- or hyper-nasality or changes in intonation. All movements are dependent upon the action of muscles of which only some are under voluntary control. Muscles are used for breathing, walking and performing manoeuvres with the hands; those concerned with articulation clearly play an important part in the production of speech. Muscles form 80% of the body weight and there are over 200 named ones in the body. Each muscle consists of bundles of microscopic muscle fibres which are capable of contracting and relaxing under nervous control mediated by biochemical means. By virtue of the attachments of muscles, shortening of the fibres resulting from their contraction produces movement. Individual muscles are supplied by the cranial or spinal nerves which form the necessary connections with the brain stem or spinal cord respectively.

The nervous impulses which control movement are transmitted along the motor pathway extending from the cerebral cortex to the peripheral nerve supplying the muscles. The parts extending from the motor nuclei of the cranial nerves along their nerve fibres to the neuro-muscular junction (the motor end plate) and from the anterior horn cells in the spinal cord along the fibres of the spinal nerves to their motor end plates constitute the *lower motor neurones* (L.M.N.).

Each nerve fibre supplies a large number of muscle fibres, the number varying with the type of muscle, e.g. the average limb muscle will have about one nerve fibre supplying 100 muscle fibres, whereas in the external ocular muscles the ratio is approximately 1 to 4. The nerve fibre together with the muscle fibres it supplies is called a 'motor unit'. The nerve cells of the lower motor neurones (i.e. the motor nuclei of the cranial nerves and the anterior horn cells of the spinal cord) are linked to other parts of the nervous system, which help in controlling movements (see Fig. 5).

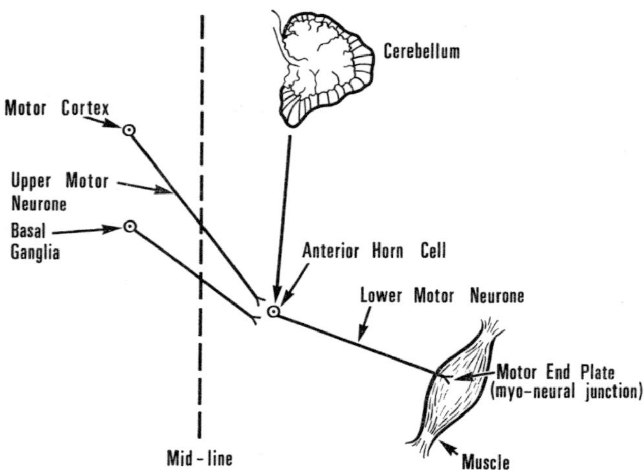

FIG. 5. Diagrammatic representation of control of muscle.

Disorders of the lower motor neurones are characterised by wasting and weakness of the muscles affected, tone is decreased leading to flaccidity, reflexes are reduced or absent, and electromyographic investigation (E.M.G.) of the nerves and the muscles supplied by them show characteristic changes. In some cases of lower motor neurone involvement, particularly when there is active degeneration of the anterior horn cells, the affected muscles show spontaneous small contractions—fasciculation. This can also be shown on the electromyogram and is a typical feature of motor neurone disease (see page 42).

Disorders may affect any part of the upper motor neurones from its origin in the motor cortex to its termination in the synapse with the corresponding cell of the lower motor neurone (Fig. 3). There is usually no wasting or just a little due to disuse. The muscles supplied by the affected nerves become weak or paralysed, the tendon reflexes on the affected side being exaggerated and the plantar response becomes extensor. Paralysis may involve one limb (monoplegia), one half of the body (hemiplegia), both legs (paraplegia) or all four limbs (quadriplegia).

The main differences between the clinical signs of the upper and lower motor neurone lesions are summarised in Table 1.

TABLE 1. Summary of the differences between upper and lower motor neuron lesions.

	U.M.N.	L.M.N.
Distribution of weakness	whole limb or part	groups of muscles
Tone	increased	decreased
Reflexes	increased	decreased
Plantar response	extensor	absent or flexor
Wasting	absent	present
Fasciculation	absent	present in some

Most of the motor nuclei of the cranial nerves in the brain stem have bilateral U.M.N. representation, i.e. cortico-bulbar fibres from both cerebral hemispheres (some crossed and some uncrossed) form synapses with the motor nuclei on each side. Part of the motor nucleus of the facial nerve supplying the muscles of the *lower* part of the face does not have bilateral representation, i.e. it is controlled only by the crossed cortico-bulbar fibres originating from the face area of the opposite cerebral hemisphere. If these upper motor neurones are damaged, there will be weakness of the muscles in the lower part of the face on the opposite side; this is in contrast to the *upper* part of the face in which power of the muscles is largely maintained because they are controlled by a different part of the nucleus of the facial nerve which does have bilateral representation, function being preserved by the uncrossed fibres originating from the unaffected cerebral hemisphere. In these cases the facial weakness is more obvious with emotional movements than with volition.

A tumour or haemorrhage damaging the upper motor neurones in one cerebral hemisphere produces paralysis on the opposite side of the body. This will principally affect the lower part of the face, arm and leg, producing the upper motor neurone signs mentioned, movements of the muscles which have bilateral representation being unaffected, (i.e. movements of the eyes, jaws, upper part of the face, soft palate, neck and tongue).

Synapse

A synapse is the gap between the termination of one nerve fibre and the cell body of another neurone, around which there is an area of electrical excitability highly sensitive to the chemical substances responsible for the transmission and modification of impulses. Nerve fibres from the cerebellum and brain stem, the basal ganglia (of the extra-pyramidal system) also terminate at the synapses of the L.M.N. and the impulses interact with those conveyed by the U.M.N. Co-ordinate muscular action, tone and posture depend upon the integrated functions of all these fibre tracts (see Fig. 5).

NEUROLOGICAL CAUSES OF DYSARTHRIA

The neurological causes of dysarthria are classified according to which part of the neuromuscular system is affected. The disorders may thus involve:

(1) Muscles
(2) Lower motor neurones
(3) Upper motor neurones
(4) Extra-pyramidal system
(5) Cerebellum and its connections
(6) Cerebral cortex (motor speech area)

and will be described under these headings.

DISORDERS OF MUSCLES

All primary disorders of muscles are referred to as 'myopathies'. They are characterised by weakness and wasting of the muscles affected with reduction or loss of associated tendon reflexes. The electrical reactions of the muscle tested by electromyography are abnormal.

The different diseases have a predilection for certain groups of muscles and can be recognised by the particular pattern and distribution of the muscles affected. Whether speech is involved will depend upon the type and extent of the disease. The main diseases that have to be considered are:

(1) The muscular dystrophies
(2) Polymyositis
(3) Myasthenia gravis.

The chief characteristics of these diseases are indicated in Table 2.

Myasthenia gravis is thought to be due to a biochemical disorder at the myoneural junction. The contraction of muscles is normally dependent on the action of acetyl-choline, the substance liberated at the motor end-plate when an electrical discharge reaches the neuro-muscular junction. In myasthenia gravis, either insufficient acetyl-choline is produced or it is too rapidly destroyed by excess of the naturally occurring enzyme, cholinesterase. As a result of this, the muscles fatigue sooner than normal and become progressively weaker as they are used, but power usually recovers after a period of rest.

The condition may occur at any age but usually between 20 and 50 years; it is slightly more frequent in females. The commonest mode of presentation in about 80% of cases is with ocular symptoms such as double vision (diplopia) and drooping of the upper eyelid (ptosis). Not infrequently, the voice becomes fainter (dysphonic) after talking for some time and the jaw may become so weak that it has to be supported by hand. The symptoms are worse in the evenings and after using the affected muscles, and are relieved by rest.

The diagnosis is usually established by giving a test dose of tensilon intravenously; within a few seconds this blocks the activity

TABLE 2. Disorders of muscles (myopathies)

	Pathology and aetiology	Signs and symptoms		Treatment
		General	Speech	
1. Muscular dystrophies	Various types affecting different groups of muscles. Abnormalities of muscle enzymes, usually hereditary.	Weakness and wasting of affected muscles. Slow progression.	Slurred speech if articulatory muscles involved.	Nil specific.
2. Polymyositis	Inflammatory disease of muscles and sometimes skin (dermatomyositis). Usually a collagen disease, 10% associated with cancer.	Usually proximal muscles weak, painful and tender.	May be slurred and slow.	Steroids.
3. Myasthenia gravis	Biochemical disorder of neuromuscular transmission. Excessive fatiguability of muscles. 10–15% associated with tumour of thymus (thymoma).	Usually affects eye muscles causing diplopia and ptosis. Dysphagia and generalised weakness may occur.	Articulation becomes increasingly indistinct and the voice weak. Recovery following rest or injection of tensilon or prostigmine.	Prostigmine. Thymectomy.

of cholinesterase, acetyl-choline is then not destroyed so quickly and muscle power is restored temporarily. This relief lasts for a few minutes only and weakness then returns. Alternatively prostigmine can be given intramuscularly; it has the same effect after about 15 minutes and acts for about an hour. In most cases treatment is effective with prostigmine tablets taken by mouth.

DISORDERS OF LOWER MOTOR NEURONES

The lower motor neurones controlling the muscles used for articulation (as well as phonation and swallowing) form the 7th, 9th, 10th, 11th and 12th cranial nerves originating from their motor nuclei in the brain stem. These supply the muscles of the lips, palate, pharynx, larynx and tongue, and knowledge of their anatomy is required.

Seventh cranial (facial) nerve leaves the lower border of the pons on each side and passes through the skull in the facial canal in close proximity to the eighth cranial (acoustic) nerve. It emerges through the stylomastoid foramen and supplies the muscles which control facial expression, raising the eyebrows, frowning, closing the eyes, as well as the movements of the lips and mouth.

The 9th, 10th and 11th cranial nerves leave the medulla on each side and pass through the skull in the jugular foramen.

Ninth cranial (glossopharyngeal) nerve supplies only one muscle, the stylo-pharyngeus and conveys sensation from the pharynx and posterior third of the tongue including taste.

Tenth cranial (vagus) nerve supplies (a) the muscles of the palate (with the exception of the tensor palati which is supplied by the mandibular branch of the 5th nerve); (b) the muscles of the pharynx, namely the three constrictors, and the salpingo- and palato-pharyngeus, but not the stylo-pharyngeus muscle (see above); (c) the intrinsic muscles of the larynx, the external cricothyroid muscle being supplied by the external branch of the superior laryngeal nerve and the remaining intrinsic muscles of the larynx by the recurrent laryngeal nerves which have a different course on the two sides; and (d) viscera via the cardiac and gastric plexuses.

Eleventh cranial (accessory) nerve is a purely motor nerve, composed of two parts, cranial and spinal. The *cranial part* joins the vagus nerve and contributes to the functions described above. The *spinal part* arises from grey matter in the lateral part of the anterior horn of the upper 5 cervical cord segments, and forms a trunk which passes upwards through the foramen magnum; it briefly makes contact with the cranial part of the accessory nerve and the vagus, and with them passes out of the skull again through the jugular foramen. It then supplies the sterno-mastoid and trapezius muscles.

Twelfth cranial (hypoglossal) nerve leaves the lower part of the medulla on each side and passes through the skull in the hypoglossal foramen. It traverses the deep structures of the neck and supplies the muscles of the tongue.

Disorders of lower motor neurones causing dysarthria are divided into two groups, depending on whether there is involvement of the cranial nerves (7th, 9th, 10th, 11th or 12th) or of their motor nuclei in the brain stem.

A. *Disorders of cranial nerves* (7, 9, 10, 11 and 12)

(1) Polyneuritis
(2) Damage by neoplasm, goitre, aneurysm or trauma
(3) Bell's palsy.

B. *Disorders of motor nuclei in the brain stem*

(1) Poliomyelitis
(2) Motor neurone disease (progressive bulbar palsy)
(3) Syringobulbia
(4) Neoplasm.

For further details of these conditions, see Table 3, A and B. Dysarthria due to the disorders of the lower motor neurones may form part of the clinical syndrome of bulbar palsy.

BULBAR PALSY

Mechanism of production

Bulbar palsy implies that there is weakness of the muscles supplied by the cranial nerves whose motor nuclei lie in the medulla or bulb. The disease causing bulbar palsy involve either these motor nuclei, the cranial nerves themselves, their motor end plates or the muscles supplied (see Tables 2 and 3 A, B).

TABLE 3A. Disorders of lower motor neurones.
A. Involving cranial nerves 7th, 9th, 10th, 11th, 12th.

	Pathology and aetiology	Signs and symptoms		Treatment
		General	Speech	
1. Polyneuritis	Acute type following infections, occasionally glandular fever etc. Chronic cases e.g. due to diabetes and alcohol.	Symmetrical weakness and sensory changes usually starting in distal parts of limbs and 'muzzle' area of face. Spinal and cranial nerves may be affected.	Dysarthria, nasal voice and dysphonia result if the lower cranial nerves are affected due to paresis of lips, palate, pharynx, larynx and tongue.	Rest in acute stage, postural drainage or tracheostomy and assisted respiration may be necessary.
2. Damage to cranial nerves	Neoplasm Goitre Aneurysm of aorta Trauma.	Local effects dependent on the type and site of the pathological lesion.	as above.	Sometimes surgical.
3. Bell's palsy	Inflammatory or ischaemic lesion of 7th cranial (facial) nerve in stylomastoid canal. Usually recovers.	Paralysis of the facial muscles on the affected side.	Slurred speech due to unilateral facial weakness affecting muscles around the mouth.	Physiotherapy for facial muscles. Occasionally steroids or surgery.

TABLE 3B.

B. Involving motor nuclei of brain stem.

	Pathology and aetiology	Signs and symptoms		Treatment
		General	Speech	
1. Poliomyelitis	Virus infection of motor nuclei of cranial nerves in brain stem and anterior horn cells of spinal cord. Mild cases are reversible, severe irreversible.	Paresis or paralysis of limb muscles with wasting and L.M.N. signs. No sensory loss. Bulbar palsy. Respiratory paralysis.	Dysarthria, dysphonia.	As for polyneuritis.
2. Motor neurone disease	Cause unknown. Onset usually in middle age. Progressive deterioration with death usually in 2–4 years.	Progressive bulbar palsy. Wasting and fasciculation of tongue, and muscles of limbs (amyotrophy). Saliva in excess due to pharyngeal weakness with dysphagia. U.M.Ns also involved (see Table 4).	Dysarthria, articulation becomes more indistinct, labials most noticeably affected due to paresis of lips, progressive weakness of tongue impairs dental and velar sounds. Dysphonia, weakness of soft palate	Nil specific.

(**Syringomyelia**)	starting around 4th ventricle and central canal of spinal cord. Developmental disorder. Onset of symptoms usually between 20 and 40. Slowly progressive.	loss on face associated with manifestations of syringomyelia—i.e. wasting of small muscles of the hands, trophic changes etc.		sion occasionally indicated.
4. Neoplasm	Glioma—rare in brain stem, usually children.	Signs of progressive involvement of cranial nerve nuclei, often starting in the pons, may be asymmetrical.	as above.	Radiotherapy

Clinical features

The main clinical features are dysarthria, dysphagia and dysphonia with weakness and wasting of the muscles supplied by the lower cranial nerves. Weakness of elevation of the soft palate may fail to close off the nasopharynx, so that when speaking there is excessive nasality of the voice (hyper-rhinolalia) and when swallowing nasal regurgitation may occur particularly with fluids. In the progressive bulbar palsy due to motor neurone disease, fasciculation in the tongue and other muscles is a characteristic feature.

The dysarthria of bulbar palsy in which the weakness of the muscles is associated with wasting usually affects all consonants and differs from that of pseudo-bulbar palsy in which the muscle weakness is associated with spasticity.

Associated signs

There may be more generalised lower motor neurone involvement affecting the muscles of the trunk and limbs, supplied by the spinal nerves originating from the affected anterior horn cells of the spinal cord. These muscles will then also develop weakness, wasting and flaccidity with dimunition or absence of tendon reflexes.

DISORDERS OF UPPER MOTOR NEURONES

Dysarthria only results from unilateral upper motor neurone involvement if this causes severe weakness around the mouth and lips on the affected side. Otherwise disorders of upper motor neurones must be *bilateral* to cause dysarthria, and the causes can be classified as follows:

(1) Cerebral vascular lesions
(2) Motor neurone disease
(3) Congenital disorders—e.g. "spastics"
(4) Neoplasms—e.g. metastases
(5) Miscellaneous—encephalitis, degenerative diseases, severe brain injuries.

For further details of these conditions, see Table 4.

Dysarthria due to the disorders of upper motor neurones bilaterally may form part of the clinical syndrome of pseudobulbar palsy.

PSEUDOBULBAR PALSY

Mechanism of Production

Pseudobulbar palsy is not primarily a disease of the bulb but of the cortico-bulbar fibres, i.e. that part of the upper motor neurone extending from the Betz cells in the motor cortex and terminating in the brain stem at the synapses with the motor nuclei of the cranial nerves.

The term supra-bulbar palsy is sometimes used synonymously with pseudobulbar palsy; it is accurate because it implies that the fibres above the bulb are affected and that the lesion is not actually in the bulb. The term pseudobulbar palsy is preferred because it describes the clinical state resembling bulbar palsy.

The involvement of cortico-bulbar fibres must be *bilateral* to produce pseudobulbar palsy. This is because not all the cortico-bulbar fibres cross in the brain stem; some remain uncrossed and continue down on the same side. If the upper motor neurone lesion is unilateral the muscles are not obviously affected and pseudobulbar palsy will not result.

Clinical features

Dysarthria and dysphagia are the main clinical effects of pseudobulbar palsy. The tone and reflexes of the affected muscles are increased, so there is a brisk jaw jerk, spasticity of the face and exaggeration of the palatal and pharyngeal reflexes. Spasticity in the tongue makes it appear smaller.

Associated signs

In addition to the bilateral involvement of cortico-bulbar fibres, the same diseases may affect cortico-spinal fibres producing upper motor neurone signs in the trunk and limbs with weakness, spasticity (increased tone) and clonus, exaggerated tendon reflexes and extensor plantar responses. There may be impairment of voluntary control of emotional expression, and exaggeration or prolongation of normal responses, perhaps laughing and crying

TABLE 4. Disorders of upper motor neurones (BILATERALLY) causing pseudobulbar palsy.

	Pathology and aetiology	Signs and symptoms		Treatment
		General	Speech	
1. **Cerebral vascular lesions**	Arteriosclerosis. Infarction. Haemorrhage. Often associated with hypertension and heart diseases (see Chapter 12).	Often double hemiplegia. Mental condition impaired. Emotional lability. Jaw jerk increased. Spasticity of face. Dysphagia. All may improve.	Slurred indistinct articulation. Voice weak (Dysphasia as well if dominant cerebral hemisphere is affected).	Nursing care during acute stages.
2. **Motor neurone disease**	Cause unknown. Onset usually in middle age. Progressive deterioration with death usually in 2–4 years.	Spastic weakness of muscles, including face, pharynx and limbs. Jaw jerk and limb reflexes exaggerated. Dysphagia. Difficulty coughing. Respiratory distress. L.M.Ns also involved (see Table 3B).	Spastic type of dysarthria and dysphonia.	Nil specific.

3. Congenital disorders	Environmental and genetic causes. Cerebral palsy (see Chapter 14).	Spastic weakness of limbs, sometimes with 'scissors gait'. Mental retardation and epilepsy often but not invariably associated.	Dysarthria, may be staccato or explosive. Tongue spastic. Specific language defects.	Muscular education with relaxation exercises and physiotherapy. Speech therapy and special schooling important.
4. Neoplasms	Metastases in both cerebral hemispheres, most commonly from primary malignant tumour in lung (see Chapter 11).	Dependent on localisation of deposits. Raised intra-cranial pressure, i.e. headache, vomiting and papilloedema.	Dysarthria (may be dysphasia as well).	Radiotherapy in selected cases.
5. Miscellaneous	Encephalitis. Degenerative diseases. Severe brain injuries.	Mental confusion. Spasticity in limbs. Epilepsy.	Dysarthria. Dysphonia.	Nursing care, sometimes steroids. Speech therapy and physiotherapy, in suitable cases.

for no apparent reason, causing considerable distress and embarrassment.

Causes of pseudobulbar palsy

The commonest cause of pseudobulbar palsy is *cerebro-vascular disease* involving both cerebral hemispheres. Typically there is a history of a stroke, i.e. infarction or haemorrhage in one cerebral hemisphere (see Chapter 12) followed by recovery and later a second stroke affecting the other cerebral hemisphere. The cortico-bulbar fibres may have been damaged on the side of the first stroke, but without overt signs because of their bilateral representation. Whether or not there is a residual hemiplegia, the defect of the cortico-bulbar fibres will not be apparent until the second stroke involves the opposite cerebral hemisphere whereupon pseudo-bulbar palsy results.

Motor neurone disease can also cause pseudobulbar palsy by progressive involvement of cortico-bulbar fibres bilaterally. This disease may also cause progressive involvement of cortico-spinal tracts, the motor nuclei of the cranial nerves and the anterior horn cells more or less symmetrically. Thus in some cases, there will be combined features of both bulbar and pseudobulbar palsy, as well as amyotrophy and upper motor neurone signs in the limbs.

Pseudobulbar palsy may also result from *congenital defects*, such as faulty development of the cortico-bulbar fibres and birth trauma. If cortico-spinal fibres are also involved, then the pseudobulbar palsy is associated with spasticity of the limbs.

There are other causes of pseudobulbar palsy, such as bilateral *tumours of the brain* (see Chapter 11) e.g. secondary deposits (metastases) in both cerebral hemispheres.

Various combinations of these conditions can cause pesudobulbar palsy; for example a patient may have a tumour in one cerebral hemisphere, and a stroke affecting the other; one hemisphere may be damaged by a head injury, and the other by a vascular lesion or tumour. Pseudobulbar palsy results *only* from *bilateral* lesions of the cortico-bulbar pathways and the signs are those of upper motor neurone involvement.

CHAPTER 7

DYSARTHRIA II

DISORDERS OF THE EXTRAPYRAMIDAL SYSTEM

The Basal Ganglia

These are nuclei of grey matter lying deep in the substance of each cerebral hemisphere. They include the globus pallidus, putamen and caudate nuclei (corpus striatum), substantia nigra, subthalamic nucleus (corpus Luysii) and the red nucleus in the upper part of the midbrain. The basal ganglia are the nuclei of the extra-pyramidal system. Via connections with other parts of the central nervous system, they help to control movement, tone and posture. The mechanism of control is complicated, but diseases of the extra-pyramidal system result in involuntary movements and disorders of tone and posture. Involuntary movements include tremor as seen in Parkinson's disease, chorea, athetosis and ballismus.

The disorders of extra-pyramidal system which can cause dysarthria are:

(1) Parkinson's disease
(2) Chorea—Sydenham's (rheumatic)
—Huntington's
(3) Congenital choreo-athetosis
(4) Wilson's disease (hepato-lenticular degeneration).

The *tremor of Parkinsonism* is typically coarse and rhythmical, more marked at rest than on action. It usually starts in one hand and is classically described as 'pillrolling'. There may be poverty of movement (hypokinesia) as well as slowness and stiffness of movements which cause a mask-like expression of the face, and

TABLE 5. Disorders of the extra-pyramidal system.

Disease	Pathology and aetiology	Signs and symptoms		Treatment
		General	Speech	
1. **Parkinsonism**	(a) Idiopathic—paralysis agitans. (b) Post-encephalitic. (c) Arteriosclerotic. (d) Toxic: 1. carbon monoxide 2. manganese 3. anoxia 4. drugs, e.g. largactil.	Cogwheel rigidity. Tremor, 'pill-rolling' movement of the hands. Shuffling, festinant gait. Expressionless face. Excessive salivation, drooling.	Slow with thin, feeble, monotonous voice. Dysphonia. Dysarthria. Rapid repetitions (palilalia).	Drugs, e.g. artane and L-dopa. Neurosurgery, e.g. stereotactic thalamotomy.
2. **Chorea**	(a) Sydenham's chorea, may be associated with rheumatic fever	Choreiform movements. Grimacing, fidgeting and dropping things. Other manifestations of rheumatic fever.	Speech hesitant and jerky. Dysarthria due to jerky movements of articulatory and respiratory muscles.	Rest. Sedation. Salicylates.
	(b) Huntington's chorea Age of onset 30–50 years. Familial. Progressive and fatal.	Choreiform movements. Dementia.	Dysarthria becoming unintelligible.	No specific treatment.

3. **Athetosis.** (choreo athetosis)	(a) Agenesis or dysgenesis (b) Anoxia at birth (c) Severe neo-natal jaundice—'kernicterus'.	Writhing, purposeless, involuntary movements.	Explosive and indistint. Tongue lacks voluntary control and is overactive. Facial grimacing with continual movements of lips. Irregular spasmodic contractions of diaphragm and other respiratory muscles giving jerky quality to voice.	Motor re-education with special schooling.
4. **Hepato-lenticular degeneration.** (Wilson's disease)	Familial, age of onset 10–26 years. Deficiency of copper-binding protein, caeruloplasmin, leading to deposition of copper in corpus striatum and liver.	Muscular rigidity and involuntary movements. Cirrhosis of liver causing jaundice. Deposition of copper in the cornea of the eye forming Kayser-Fleischer ring.	Rigidity of muscles affecting articulation and phonation.	Chelating agents e.g. penicillamine.

rigidity of cog-wheel type in the limbs. There are usually defects of fine and associated movements. The posture is often stooped and the limbs slightly flexed, the legs shuffling along so that the gait appears hurried or festinant with 'marche à petits pas'. There is no wasting, the reflexes are unaffected and the plantar responses flexor.

The speech in Parkinsonism is characteristically monotonous. Rigidity of the muscles of the larynx makes the voice weak and feeble, i.e. dysphonic. Involvement of the muscles used for articulation results in dysarthria. Speech may also be affected in a way comparable to the festinant gait, i.e. words following each other faster and faster, and the same phrase may be repeated over and over again (palilalia). In some patients, excessive salivation or difficulty in swallowing causes dribbling and slobbering which may be exaggerated by the tremor of mouth and tongue.

Chorea usually affects the peripheral parts of the limbs and causes jerky movements whilst the movements of *athetosis* are writhing, and both are purposeless and involuntary.

A lesion of the subthalamic nucleus on one side results in *hemiballismus* affecting the limbs on the other side of the body. Ballismic movements are involuntary, throwing, purposeless movements, affecting particularly the proximal parts of the limbs, often flinging the limb around violently.

Chorea and athetosis cause jerkiness of speech, sometimes with an explosive dysarthria due to sudden involuntary movements affecting respiratory muscles, larynx or mouth, and in severe cases speech is unintelligible.

Further details of the diseases of the extra-pyramidal system are given in Table 5.

DISORDERS OF THE CEREBELLUM

The cerebellum consists of right and left cerebellar hemispheres joined in the midline by the vermis. Each cerebellar hemisphere is connected to the corresponding side of the brain stem by three cerebellar peduncles: (1) superior (brachium conjunctivum), (2) middle (brachium pontis) and (3) inferior (restiform body).

The cerebellum and its connections control the co-ordination of movements and influence muscle tone. There are important connections with the vestibular mechanisms and cranial nerve nuclei concerned with movements of the muscles of the eyes and neck. Because of this, the maintenance of balance and co-ordination of movements are dependent upon the integrity of the cerebellum and its connections.

Disturbances of cerebellar function will result in defects of co-ordination and balance, and affect speech muscles as well as the muscles of the eyes, neck, trunk and limbs.

CEREBELLAR SIGNS

Since the main cerebellar fibres are uncrossed, defects of one cerebellar hemisphere will cause inco-ordination in the muscles on the same side of the body; bilateral cerebellar involvement causes generalised inco-ordination of all limbs, and lesions confined to the vermis affect co-ordination of the trunk and neck muscles.

Inco-ordination affecting the upper limbs is seen as 'intention tremor' i.e. tremor on movement; other signs include difficulty performing rapidly repetitive or alternating movements (dysdiadokokinesis), poor control of the range of movements (dysmetria) and clumsiness. Clinical tests used to demonstrate these defects include maintenance of posture of outstretched hands and finger-nose-finger test.

Inco-ordination affects balance and causes unsteadiness when walking (ataxia) so that the patient veers to one side and tends to sway or stumble. The maintenance of posture and control of movements of the muscles of the neck may be affected so that the head appears to jerk or waver irregularly (titubation).

Since co-ordination of eye movements is dependent upon the connections between the oculo-motor, vestibular and cerebellar pathways, cerebellar lesions are often associated with nystagmus, i.e. a rhythmical involuntary jerking movement of the eyes, usually elicited by asking the patient to look to one side, but sometimes occurring spontaneously when looking straight ahead.

The muscles of articulation may also be affected by cerebellar inco-ordination, resulting in ataxic dysarthria. In mild forms, this begins as slurring of speech and the pronunciation of consonants is particularly difficult. Speech becomes slow and thick 'as if there is something in the mouth' and slurring and jerkiness may be combined. Due to poor control of rhythm, there is a tendency to pronounce each syllable as if it is a separate word (scanning speech) and to put the emphasis on the wrong syllables, some being pronounced too loudly and others too softly (staccato speech). In severe cases speech may become explosive and unintelligible, eventually with complete inability to articulate (anarthria).

DISEASES OF THE CEREBELLUM

(1) Multiple (disseminated) sclerosis.
(2) Hereditary ataxias, e.g. Friedreich's.
(3) Degenerations, e.g. idiopathic, carcinomatous.
(4) Metabolic and toxic disorders, e.g. hypothyroidism, drugs (alcohol etc.).
(5) Congenital disorders, e.g. dysgenesis.
(6) Miscellaneous, e.g. vascular lesions, abscess, neoplasms.

Multiple Sclerosis

The axon (nerve fibre) is surrounded by a tube or sheath of myelin and the disease, multiple sclerosis, is characterised by patches or plaques of demyelination. The cause of the disease is unknown, as is the explanation for the patchy distribution of plaques. Initially there is an inflammatory or allergic reaction around the plaques, which usually subsides spontaneously and may be followed by remyelination. The scar formation in the nervous system is called gliosis and hardening of the plaques with time results in patches of sclerosis. The plaques seem to have a predilection for certain parts of the nervous system, in particular the optic nerves, the cerebellum, brain stem and spinal cord. They may also occur throughout the cerebral hemispheres, not infrequently in the later stages of the disease.

The disease usually starts in young adults between the ages of 20 and 45 but occasionally in the late teens, and less frequently in middle age. Females are affected more than males in the ratio of 3:2 and the incidence of the disease varies in different parts of the world, being commoner in temperate climates. In England the

TABLE 6. Disorders of the cerebellum.

Disease	Pathology and aetiology	Signs and symptoms: General	Signs and symptoms: Speech	Treatment
1. **Multiple sclerosis**	Plaques of demyelination scattered throughout the C.N.S. and optic nerves. Irregular course of relapses and remissions. Onset 20–45 years. Females more commonly than males.	Optic neuritis. Diplopia. Vertigo. Cerebellar signs: Intention tremor Nystagmus Ataxia. Sensory disturbances. U.M.N. (pyramidal) signs.	Slurred. Scanning. Staccato. Dysphasia very rare.	Avoidance of fatigue. A.C.T.H. for acute relapses. Physiotherapy.
2. **Hereditary ataxias**	Friedreich's disease is the commonest affecting cerebellum, cerebellar connections, pyramidal tracts and posterior columns. Associated skeletal deformities (pes cavus, kyphoscoliosis) and cardiac abnormalities. Onset in adolescence, slowly progressive.	Cerebellar signs; U.M.N. (pyramidal) signs; posterior column signs: loss of position and vibration sense. Ataxia predominates due to cerebellar incoordination and loss of position sense: absent knee jerks and ankle jerks with bilateral extensor plantar responses.	Slow. Slurred. Explosive.	Aids for co-ordination. Physiotherapy, balancing exercises.

TABLE 6. Disorders of the cerebellum—*continued.*

Disease	Pathology and aetiology	Signs and symptoms: General	Signs and symptoms: Speech	Treatment
3. **Degenerations**	(a) Idiopathic, cerebellar atrophy. Onset later in life after 40 or 50. Slowly progressive course. No associated skeletal or cardiac disorders.	as above.	as above.	as above.
	(b) Carcinomatous degeneration usually associated with carcinoma of the bronchus. Not due to metastases in the cerebellum.	Ataxia. Cough, shadow on chest X-ray (sometimes neuropathy as well).	Dysarthria.	Nil specific. Removal of primary growth if operable, or radiotherapy.
4. **Metabolic and toxic disorders.**	Hypothyroidism. Alcoholism.	Myxoedema. Liver disease.	Husky voice. Dysarthria.	Thyroid. Avoidance of alcohol.

5. Congenital disorders.	Agenesis or dysgenesis of cerebellum.	Oro-facial muscles under-developed. Grimacing and drooling. Lack of control of voluntary movement and of posture.	Delayed development. Slurred, jerky.	Aids for co-ordination. Physiotherapy, balancing exercises. Speech therapy.
6. Miscellaneous.	(a) Vascular lesions, infarction, haemorrhage, often with hypertension.	Mainly ipsilateral cerebellar signs, sudden onset.	Dysarthria.	Operation for removal of intracerebellar haematoma. Nursing care. Speech therapy and physiotherapy during recovery.
	(b) Abscess, usually from otitis media (see Chapter 13). (c) Neoplasms (see Chapter 11).	Ipsilateral cerebellar signs, progressive. Raised intracranial pressure.	Dysarthria.	Antibiotics. Neurosurgery. Speech therapy and physiotherapy following operation on benign tumour or abscess.

prevalence is about 40 per 100,000 but there is a tendency for clusters of cases to occur in certain areas.

Usually the disease is characterised by relapses and remissions, so a plaque may develop first in an optic nerve causing poor vision in one eye with recovery after a few weeks. The spontaneous recovery (remission) may then be followed by another relapse e.g. a plaque in the spinal cord causing paraplegia. Plaques occur either singly in various parts of the nervous system at different times, or in crops. After each successive relapse, there tends to be less recovery and thus more severe and persistent disability. Recovery from each relapse may take several weeks or months but remissions can last for months, years or life. In about 20% of cases, the disease runs a progressive course.

The plaques involving the cerebellum or its brain stem connections cause a variety of cerebellar signs which may include nystagmus, titubation, clumsiness of the hands with intention tremor, and ataxia of gait. Speech becomes slurred, typically with a scanning or staccato type of dysarthria. Manifestations of the disease affecting other parts of the nervous system are frequently present at the same time or occur in subsequent relapses. These include visual and sensory symptoms, vertigo, loss of bladder control and upper motor neurone signs due to plaques in the spinal cord.

There is as yet no specific cure, but physiotherapy is usually advocated, and treatment with A.C.T.H. during acute relapses may enhance remission.

For further details of the disorders of the cerebellum see Table 6.

DISORDERS OF THE CEREBRAL CORTEX

Dysarthria occasionally results from lesions of the premotor area, which exerts cerebral control over the muscles of the face and those used for speech. This may be associated with motor or expressive dysphasia, and is called apraxic or cortical dysarthria. It results from the same pathological conditions which cause motor dysphasia (see Chapter 5) and from general paralysis of the insane (see page 99).

CHAPTER 8

DYSPHONIA

Dysphonia is weakness or hoarseness of the voice due to any lesion interfering with the laryngeal mechanism which governs voice production. There are a variety of non-neurological causes, the commonest of which is a sore throat with inflammation of the larynx (laryngitis). Hysteria is probably the next most common cause. This is a functional disturbance without structural defect, often a reaction to an emotional disturbance, particularly in females. These patients usually just whisper and the lack of any true laryngeal disorder is usually evident as they can cough normally. Sudden spontaneous recovery takes place when psychological equilibrium is restored.

Patients with a tracheostomy are aphonic as the tube in the trachea prevents the expired air from reaching the larynx. Tumours and local lesions of the larynx cause dysphonia and the voice tends to become deep and husky in patients with hypothyroidism (myxoedema).

The Neuromuscular Causes of Dysphonia

The mechanism of phonation is dependent on the muscles of the vocal cords supplied by the 10th cranial (vagus) nerves (see Chapter 6). The adductors and tensors of the vocal cords contract on phonation and the abductors on inspiration. The vocal cords can be viewed by laryngoscopy and weakness of one or both results in dysphonia.

Dysphonia, like dysarthria, may be caused by the muscle diseases shown in Table 2, and by the lower motor neurone disorders shown in Table 3A when these involve the vagus nerve. The recurrent laryngeal branches of the vagus are particularly prone to damage in the neck and chest by:

(1) surgery—during thyroidectomy.
(2) carcinoma of the thyroid.
(3) carcinoma of the bronchus and malignant mediastinal growths.
(4) aortic aneurysm.

A unilateral recurrent laryngeal nerve lesion causes paralysis of the vocal cord; the resulting weakness of the voice may be slight and transient due to compensatory movement by the opposite vocal cord. The abductors are always affected before the adductors (Semon's law) and therefore paralysis of adduction cannot occur without paralysis of abduction. Total bilateral paralysis of the vocal cords causes complete aphonia so that the patient can only whisper. Partial lesions causing bilateral abductor palsies produce laryngeal stridor (a harsh sound from the larynx) during inspiration.

The proximal part of the vagus nerve may be involved in the 'jugular foramen syndrome' in which the 9th, 10th and 11th cranial nerves are affected on one side. This may be caused by lesions at the base of the skull, such as a carcinoma spreading from the nasopharynx. The diseases involving the nuclei of the vagus in the medulla are shown in Table 3B, and dysphonia is part of the syndrome of bulbar palsy, as has been described in Chapter 6.

Dysphonia is also one of the features of pseudo-bulbar palsy, resulting from the disorders of upper motor neurones (bilaterally) as shown in Table 4.

Of the extra-pyramidal disorders shown in Table 5, dysphonia occurs most commonly in Parkinsonism, when the voice tends to be weak and monotonous. Dysphonia is rarely associated with cerebellar lesions, unless these involve the brain stem as well.

CHAPTER 9

DEMENTIA

Dementia means deterioration of intellectual functions, so that there is impairment of memory, intelligence and a wide variety of aptitudes and accomplishments. The term has usually been used to imply an irreversible state as the conditions causing dementia were nearly always progressive or untreatable. This is no longer invariably the case, since several causes of dementia can now be treated effectively e.g. benign intracranial tumours, neurosyphilis and Vitamin B12 deficiency. Early diagnosis of these treatable conditions is important as the degree of recovery depends largely on how early treatment is started. All patients with dementia therefore require investigation to establish the cause as soon as possible.

Dementia must be distinguished from amentia, which is the failure or impairment of intellectual development. Mental and intellectual faculties are dependent on the integrated and selective functions of the millions of cells in the cerebral cortex. The greatest degree of *learning* ability is in youth although, with experience and training, memory patterns and skills are established and judgement improves. During middle life, the cells of the cerebral cortex begin to dwindle, probably by more than a 100,000 each day. This is part of the natural process of ageing (physiological senescence) so that most old people do not have the same intellectual capacity as when they were young, the earliest sign being loss of memory for recent events with a tendency to become forgetful of names. Physiological senescence and senile dementia are not synonymous as dementia implies a pathological process.

If intellectual deterioration occurs before the age of 65, the term *presenile dementia* is used, but this serves only to indicate the relatively early age of onset as the pathological causes may be the same as in the elderly.

In any patient with dementia—whatever the cause—speech may be affected, but vocabulary may be retained until quite late in the illness. Although speech therapy will not help if there is a significant degree of dementia, it is important to be aware of the different types of altered speech observed and the pathological processes of the brain which interfere with the mental faculties.

Causes of Dementia

Dementia is not a diagnosis but a manifestation (cf: dysphasia and hemiplegia) of various diseases. The underlying cause has to be established, particularly so that the potentially reversible disorders are not overlooked; the classification shown in Table 7 is suggested.

TABLE 7. Causes of dementia.

Metabolic Disorders
- Deficiency of Vitamin B_1 (Korsakoffs' psychosis, Wernicke's encephalopathy)
  - Vitamin B_2 (Pellagra)
  - Vitamin B_{12}
- Hypothyroidism
- Hypoglycaemia
- Hepatic and renal failure
- Drugs, e.g. barbiturates, alcohol, bromides arsenic, lead, mercury
- Cerebral anoxia, e.g. following cardiac arrest
- Lipidoses

Degenerative Diseases
- Alzheimer's, Pick's
- Huntington's chorea
- Jakob—Creutzfeldt disease (? due to slow virus)

Infections (see Chapter 13)
- Neurosyphilis

Hydrocephalus (see Chapter 14)
- Obstructive, Communicating

Tumours (see Chapter 11)
- e.g. of frontal lobes and corpus callosum

Trauma
- Brain injuries
- 'Punch drunk' syndrome
- Chronic subdural haematoma

The disruption of mental functions is usually generalised (global dementia) and includes deterioration of intelligence, memory, behaviour and personality. Deficits can also be selective, so that formal intelligence may be preserved yet serious lapses of judgement occur. The development of slovenliness may occasionally be an important early feature of dementia, but there is usually failure of memory and of the power of reasoning, lack of retention or recall, and loss of learning ability.

Differentiation from psychosis, particularly depression, and occasionally schizophrenia may be difficult; focal cerebral lesions which cause frontal lobe disinhibition, dysphasia and parietal lobe syndromes with apraxia must also be distinguished.

Patients who complain that they have to write notes as they are unable to remember things, usually do not have any serious disease. Their subjective forgetfulness may not be confirmed by tests and may be due to an anxiety state or neurosis, often being associated with headache and lack of concentration. The patient with organic dementia in contrast, conceals or is unaware of his disability and, lacking insight and judgement, may have to be persuaded by friends or relatives to consult a doctor.

Patients with dementia may be dysphasic or depressed as well. If the dementia is severe, disorientation in time and place occurs, sometimes accompanied by delusions and hallucinations. In advanced cases, there may be epileptic attacks and a variety of neurological signs, often with incontinence. In some, there is apathy and withdrawal whereas in others, there is a general motor restlessness, confusion, emotional lability, psychotic and anti-social behaviour. The presenting features often seem to be dependent more on the pre-morbid personality than the pathological process.

Examination of the Mental State

It is necessary to observe general behaviour, for example, relationship to other people and the response to situations and the surroundings.

Tests for memory and intellectual deterioration should include the assessment of orientation in space and time, simple arithmetical tests, such as 100 minus 7, sentence repetition, and tests of general knowledge. Obviously these tests need to be geared to the intellectual background of the individual patient.

The patient's method of speaking as well as the content should be observed and sometimes taped, particularly spontaneous talk, which may be hesitant, slow, or discursive with sudden changes of topic.

The patient's mood and the presence of delusions or hallucinations should be noted, as well as whether the patient is orientated as to his own name, identity, place, time and date.

Memory for both recent and more remote experiences can also be assessed as can the grasp of general information, insight and judgement. The patient should be asked to write something in his own time, for example a brief account of a day in his life.

The Babcock sentence, 'There is one thing a nation must have to be rich and great, and that is a large, secure supply of wood', is a useful test. It is repeated alternately by the examiner and patient until the patient says it perfectly. Normally this is achieved within two or three attempts; failure after several attempts is indicative of dementia. Gross perseveration of an error is typical of an organic intellectual loss, and fragmentary repetition is suggestive of a language defect. Gross variability in response is often characteristic of psychoneurosis, (Zangwill, 1943). The explanation of simple proverbs is another useful test.

Types of Demented Speech

Speech can be described in several ways e.g. phonetic, phonemic, linguistic, syntactic or semantic. Patients with dementia show poverty of speech so that in severe cases the patient is inaccessible. Although all forms of language—speaking, writing and reading are affected, expressive vocabulary of speech is most affected, a larger vocabulary being retained in writing and most with reading. There is difficulty in retaining series but, unlike aphasic patients, paraphasia, neologisms and portmanteaux words do not occur. Names for objects are often not completely accurate although they may have a close association. Interjections are rarely used although speech can be exclamatory. Speech is simplified consisting of statements, descriptions or requests, often of no importance.

It has been found that the ratio between the numbers of verbs and adjectives used varies, as in neurotics, and there is also variation in the length of sentences and punctuation. The frequency of the pronoun 'I' is also of interest: used in 5 % of words over a telephone by a normal person it is used in ·01 % in technical speech. Both in dementia and aphasia sentences are started but not finished (apotheosis) and there is filling in with unnecessary additions (paralogisms). Perseveration is extremely common; words are used normally but then reiterated (contamination) and this is also seen in writing (echographia). Echolalia is found in dementia as well as aphasia. In presenile dementias such as Pick's and Alzheimer's disease, speech is slow and there may be interpolation of the 's' and 't' sounds, and the voice also tends to become higher-pitched.

A demented patient has difficulty in understanding quick or noisy speech. Gesture, gesticulation, mime and mimicry may all be impaired, possibly in part due to slowness of movements (akinesia). The term *alogia* has been used for the impoverishment of speech in dementia; this differs from the purely communicative defects of dysphasia, which is due to a local cortical lesion of the specific area of the brain concerned with speech.

CHAPTER 10

EPILEPSY

About 4 or 5 per thousand of the adult population suffer from epilepsy so that in England and Wales there are approximately a quarter of a million epileptics. Epilepsy is one of the important manifestations of brain disease and epileptic attacks may occasionally cause transient disturbances of speech. The study of epilepsy is particularly helpful in understanding brain function.

The term epilepsy is used to describe recurrent disturbances of consciousness, movement, feeling or behaviour which are primarily cerebral in origin. Epilepsy is called *idiopathic* when the cause is not known, and *symptomatic* if due to local or diffuse disease. Convulsions can also result from fainting due to a fall in blood pressure (syncope), or a fall in blood sugar (hypoglycaemia) or in blood calcium (hypocalcaemia); the diagnosis in these cases depends on the nature of the underlying systemic disorder.

Epileptic attacks are paroxysmal, repetitive, usually stereotyped and cease spontaneously. The susceptibility or threshold to fits varies in different individuals, and may vary in the same individual at different times. Genetic or constitutional factors influence the liability to develop epilepsy, some brains being more susceptible. There is a wide range of factors which provoke fits.

TABLE 8. Factors provoking fits.

Hyperventilation
Photic and other reflex stimuli
Stress, anxiety, depression, sleep
Other metabolic factors
e.g. overhydration, premenstrual state,
hypoglycaemia, hypoxia, fever,
withdrawal of drugs, etc.
Structural brain lesions—diffuse and focal.

The threshold for fits is lowered by hyperventilation and photic stimulation and both these are used routinely during recording of the electroencephalogram (E.E.G.); other metabolic disturbances may have the same effect. Even in a healthy person a potent stimulus, e.g. an electric shock or analeptic drug will produce a convulsion. The list of provoking factors includes structural brain lesions, such as a cerebral tumour, abscess, or penetrating brain wound, but less than 50% of patients with these lesions develop epilepsy. This suggests that there are inhibiting factors preventing clinical attacks, as does the fact that a small proportion of people have E.E.G.s with epileptic activity, yet do not have fits. Considering the enormous amount of electrical activity in the brain, it is surprising that epilepsy is not more common.

AETIOLOGY

(a) *Idiopathic:* When the pathological cause of attacks is not known, the term idiopathic epilepsy is used. This may be due to disturbances of cell metabolism that cannot be defined by present techniques of investigation. However the E.E.G. in idiopathic epilepsy typically shows paroxysms of abnormal generalised excessive electrical discharges, probably originating centrally, either from structures deep in the cerebral hemispheres or from the reticular substance of the brain stem. This type of idiopathic epilepsy is also called centrencephalic epilepsy. Some factors predisposing to the development of idiopathic epilepsy are genetically determined (i.e. inherited) and account for the familial incidence of epilepsy. Idiopathic epileptic attacks usually begin between the ages of 2 and 20, although the onset is sometimes later.

Epilepsy can also result from defects of development or damage to the brain before birth, i.e. while the foetus is still in utero, or from injury to the brain during parturition.

(b) *Symptomatic:* Epilepsy, if not idiopathic, is a symptom of a cerebral lesion occurring in a patient with an inborn susceptibility. There are many causes of symptomatic epilepsy, some of which are shown in Table 9. Focal attacks in adults are nearly always indicative of symptomatic epilepsy. Any form of epilepsy developing after the age of 20 is referred to as 'epilepsy of late onset' to indicate that it may be symptomatic and requires special investigation. Only about 20% of these cases do in fact have a cerebral tumour, and some of the remainder will turn out to have idiopathic epilepsy in spite of the relatively late age of onset. Epilepsy—like headache—should be regarded as a symptom and not a single disease entity.

TABLE 9. Aetiology of epilepsy

IDIOPATHIC	Centrencephalic Cryptogenic
SYMPTOMATIC	Tumours Infective, e.g. encephalitis abscess neurosyphilis Cerebral infarction Angioma Trauma Toxic and degenerative diseases Metabolic disorders, e.g. hypoglycaemia uraemia liver failure

CLASSIFICATION OF EPILEPTIC ATTACKS

There are many different types of epilepsy and, quite apart from the variety of causes, as mentioned in the preceding paragraphs, epileptic attacks may be classified according to (1) the clinical features, and (2) the E.E.G. findings; these should be correlated when possible.

TABLE 10. Classification of epileptic attacks.

1. GENERALISED	(a) grand mal (b) petit mal (c) status epilepticus
2. FOCAL	(a) Jacksonian (b) temporal lobe (c) epilepsia partialis continuans

The two main types of epileptic attacks are (1) generalised and (2) focal.

1. GENERALISED EPILEPTIC ATTACKS

These are divided into (a) grand mal and (b) petit mal, names given by French neurologists who first described them.

(a) Grand mal

A grand mal attack produces sudden loss of consciousness with or without a warning. The warning or aura is transient, lasts only a few seconds and ranges from a vague feeling of faintness or giddiness to a variety of phenomena depending on the part of the cerebral cortex in which the discharge begins. The aura is followed by loss of consciousness, and the patient may fall and injure himself. There is often a sudden cry due to the involuntary expulsion of air through the closed glottis indicating the start of the *tonic phase*, i.e. sustained contraction of the body with the arms and legs held rigidly in flexion or extension. During this stage the tongue may be bitten, the patient makes gurgling, groaning or choking sounds and becomes cyanosed from asphyxia, frothing at the mouth. The tonic phase lasts for about ½ minute and is followed by the *clonic phase*, i.e. alternating contractions of the extensors and flexors of the limb muscles causing rhythmical repetitive jerking movements, i.e. convulsions. This phase usually lasts for a few minutes and during this stage incontinence of urine (involuntary micturition) may take place. This is followed by the *post-ictal state* when the patient may complain of headache, muscular pains and nausea and there is a period of confusion or sleep lasting from a few minutes to hours; sometimes actions are performed without being remembered (automatism). Not all grand mal seizures follow the same pattern, for example, the clonic phase may be very short or absent without convulsive movements or there may merely be a short bout of muscular twitching.

The E.E.G. in idiopathic grand mal typically shows paroxysms of high voltage discharges bilaterally and synchronously from both cerebral hemispheres. Grand mal attacks may thus have an idiopathic (centrencephalic) basis, but can also be symptomatic of structural cerebral lesions.

(b) Petit mal

Petit mal attacks are characterised by a momentary absence in which the mind goes blank and the child's expression appears vacant. This lasts for a matter of a few seconds or less and the eyes usually remain open and stare. The child may feel giddy, become pale or flushed, lose the thread of conversation, drop things or even fall momentarily but recovery is rapid. These attacks can occur several times a day and when very frequent, for example 100 per day, the name *pyknolepsy* is given.

The E.E.G. in petit mal has a characteristic pattern with high voltage bilaterally synchronous discharges of spike-and-wave complexes recurring regularly at 3 cycles per second (Fig. 6d). This E.E.G. picture differentiates true petit mal from other forms of minor epilepsy where loss of consciousness is also incomplete or momentary but due to focal cerebral disturbances. Petit mal almost invariably begins in childhood and is idiopathic.

2. FOCAL EPILEPTIC ATTACKS

Focal attacks are due to a local lesion of the brain. The disturbances of brain function depend upon the situation of the lesion, and the attacks consist of transient excitatory or inhibitory phenomena. If the lesion is progressive, this will lead to permanent neurological deficits.

Focal electrical discharges can remain localised but sometimes spread over the cortex and trigger off abnormal electrical activity in contiguous areas. This spread or 'march' of epileptic activity is reflected clinically; for example, attacks may begin with tingling on the right side of the face, spread to the right hand up the right arm and down the right side of the body to the leg, possibly followed by motor phenomena with twitching or jerking movements of the muscles of the right side of the body. This indicates a spread of the electrical discharge from the face area of the sensory cortex spreading upwards over the post-central gyrus and going on to involve the motor cortex. This type of focal attack with its sequential spread or march is called *Jacksonian epilepsy* (after Hughlings Jackson). The focal discharge can spread extensively, become generalised and precipitate a grand mal attack. The aura is important because it localises the epileptogenic focus, e.g. an aura of jerking of the right leg would indicate a lesion irritating the parasagittal premotor region of the left hemisphere; an aura of a peculiar smell or taste indicates a temporal lobe lesion (see later). If there is no aura because the electrical discharge very rapidly becomes generalised with loss of consciousness, or if the patient fails to remember the aura subsequently, evidence of a focal origin may still be obtained from investigations, for example, an electrical focus may be found on the E.E.G., or a cerebral tumour or angioma demonstrated by X-rays.

Temporal Lobe Epilepsy

This is a form of focal epilepsy where attacks originate from an abnormality in the temporal lobe; if the focus lies in the temporal lobe of the dominant hemisphere there may be an aura of dysphasia. There are often disturbances of memory, e.g. the patient may feel that something is familiar when in fact he has not come across it before. He may relive experiences that occurred some time previously, seeing or doing something familiar when in fact he has not seen or done it before (déjà-vu, déjà-fait phenomena); everything may feel strange and unfamiliar when it is in fact well known to him (jamais-vu). Odd sensations known as 'dreamy states' may occur, as well as the feeling of not existing (depersonalisation and derealisation). *Uncinate attacks* consist of hallucinations of smell (olfactory) and taste (gustatory) usually lasting just a few seconds. These are due to a lesion of the uncus (the medial part of the temporal lobe); the patient is aware of a smell, often with a burning or musty nature or indescribable. With this or separately, he may experience a peculiar, indescribable or perhaps familiar taste.

Various other hallucinations also occur:—

Auditory: the impression of hearing a sound, such as bells ringing, phrases from a musical theme or a voice which may or may not be familiar.

Vertiginous: the sensation of rotatory movement, either the head spinning or the room going round and round, similar to that experienced when getting off a roundabout.

Visual: formed hallucinations of vision may consist of remembered scenes, familiar objects, places, people or faces and all sorts of fictional images; there may be distortions of visual perception with micropsia, macropsia or apparent displacement of visual objects.

If visual hallucinations consist of crude (unformed) but stereotyped phenomena, for example, various shapes or abstract patterns which are not recognisable or remembered as particular objects, or flashing lights appearing in homonymous parts of the visual fields, then the epileptogenic focus is likely to be situated more posteriorly in the temporo-occipital region, closer to the calcarine (visual) cortex.

Auras resulting from focal lesions in the temporal lobe may be less distinct consisting of abdominal sensations, sickly or sinking feelings in the stomach (visceral or epigastric aura) which pass up the body to the head and may be followed by loss of consciousness, or often an indescribable sensation in the head (cephalic aura) or disturbances of behaviour (*psychomotor attacks*). Champing or sucking movements of the mouth are also manifestations of temporal lobe attacks.

STATUS EPILEPTICUS

A series of fits occasionally follow one another rapidly so that the patient has hardly recovered from one when the process is repeated (serial epilepsy). 'Status epilepticus' occurs when the fits recur repeatedly without any intervening recovery of consciousness. This is a very dangerous condition which may prove fatal so that all such cases should be admitted to hospital for appropriate treatment as soon as possible.

Focal fits which continue unabated for long periods are referred to as *epilepsia partialis continuans*.

SPEECH DISTURBANCES IN EPILEPSY

With petit mal, the attacks may interrupt the child's normal flow of speech, he may miss something that is said to him and lose the thread of conversation during the transient period of loss of awareness.

In temporal lobe epilepsy when the focus lies in the dominant hemisphere attacks may have a dysphasic aura; with an epileptogenic lesion in any part of the speech area, the attack itself may consist only of transient dysphasia or there may be a dysphasic aura preceding a grand mal seizure. The dysphasia may consist of any of the disturbances of speech and language described in Chapter 5, and such transient dysphasia—either alone or as the aura of a grand mal attack—is of great localising value indicating that a lesion lies in the speech area of the dominant cerebral hemisphere.

Dysphasia or hemiplegia discovered for the first time *after* an epileptic attack may be the result of the epileptogenic lesion, but such signs occurring post-ictally do not always have the same localising significance as the aura, as they may be due to an inhibitory effect of the fit (Todd's paralysis). Recovery from this usually takes place within a few days.

ELECTROENCEPHALOGRAPHY

Electrical activity in the human body is a reflection of the biochemical and metabolic processes of the individual cells. The electrical impulses from the brain were originally discovered by Berger, a German psychiatrist who published his first paper in 1929. These impulses can be recorded as the sum total of electrical activity of the 10,000 million cells of the cerebral cortex. The normal record consists of alpha or Berger rhythm of 9–11 cycles per second (Fig. 6a) which comes chiefly from the occipital area. The alpha rhythm is more marked when the eyes are closed and becomes less prominent with the eyes open; this is referred to as blocking of the alpha rhythm.

Abnormalities in the E.E.G. may be generalised or focal and can be of diagnostic value. The diagnosis of epilepsy depends principally on the clinical features of the attacks but the E.E.G. may be of considerable help in differentiating different types of epilepsy.

In idiopathic (centrencephalic) epilepsy, the E.E.G. shows characteristic paroxysms of bilaterally synchronous sharp complexes of high voltage. Fig. 6c shows grand mal components and Fig. 6d spike-and-wave complexes of petit mal. These abnormalities may be provoked or exaggerated in some cases by hyperventilation, photic stimulation (flicker) and occasionally by various other special techniques.

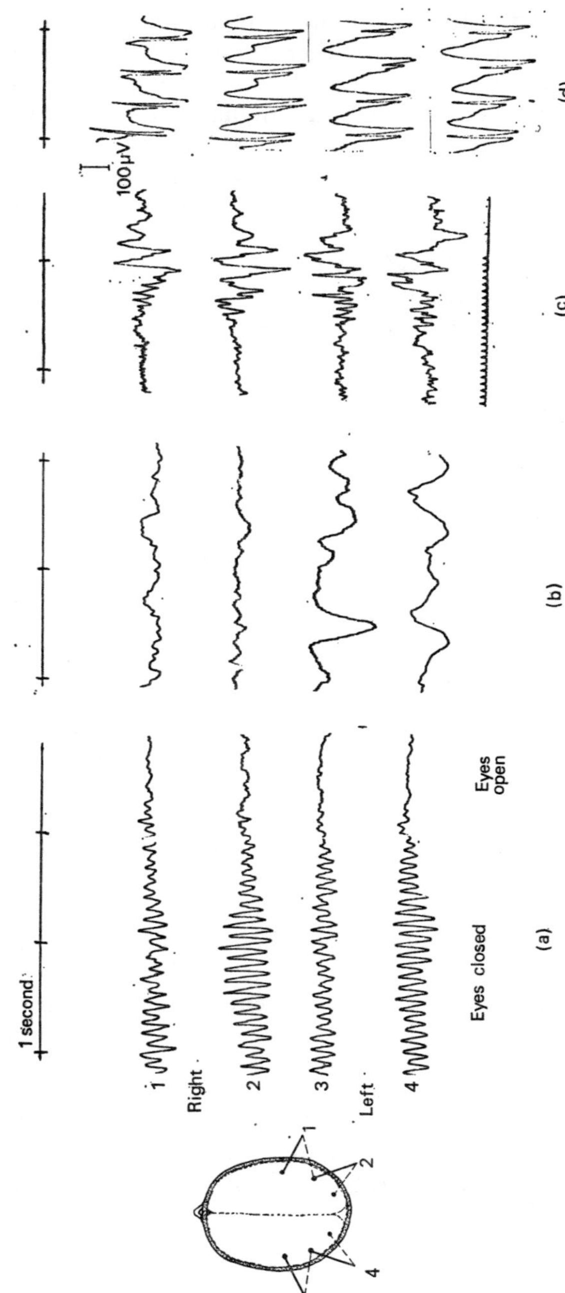

Fig. 6. Electroencephalograms. (a) Normal record; alpha rhythm blocking when eyes opened. (b) Left posterior parietal tumour; focal abnormality with slow waves. (c) Centrencephalic epilepsy; bilateral spike discharges provoked by flicker. (d) Petit mal; 3 c/s spike and wave complexes.

The usual recording between seizures leads to various diagnostic difficulties because over 10% of epileptics have a normal E.E.G and about 10% of normal people (who have never had a fit) have an abnormal E.E.G. A normal E.E.G. does not exclude idiopathic epilepsy, nor symptomatic epilepsy, since even a patient with a cerebral tumour can have a normal E.E.G. Local lesions of the brain such as tumours or abscesses may be reflected by focal abnormalities in the E.E.G. (Fig. 6b) but as a rule no conclusion regarding the pathological nature of brain lesions can be made from the E.E.G. alone.

TREATMENT OF EPILEPSY

The main drugs now used in the treatment of epilepsy are listed in Table 11.

TABLE 11. Drug treatment of epilepsy.

Petit mal	Ethosuximide (Zarontin) Troxidone (Tridione)
Grand mal and Focal	Phenobarbitone Phenytoin (Epanutin) Primidone (Mysoline)

These are the drugs usually tried first, either singly or in various combinations. They are effective in preventing attacks in a large proportion of cases. Sometimes, however, alternative or additional treatment is required and a variety of newer anticonvulsant drugs, e.g. ospolot, tegretol, benuride and valium are available.

Treatment of a grand mal attack

In order to try and prevent the tongue from being bitten something firm should be put between the teeth before they are clenched tightly; force should not be used. The patient should be prevented from doing any damage to himself or anybody else and should be allowed to lie in a space cleared of obstructions; any padding available such as cushions or blankets should be placed to prevent injury to the head and limbs during convulsions; no attempt need be made to restrain forcibly the convulsive movements. During the post-ictal phase of unconsciousness, the airway has to be kept clear, dentures should be removed, the collar loosened and the patient turned on to his side or semi-prone. Recovery usually follows without any complication; if the diagnosis of epilepsy has been established previously it is seldom necessary to call a doctor or send the patient to hospital unless an injury has been sustained in the attack and requires treatment. Medical advice should be sought for the first fit, and a series of fits in quick succession or status epilepticus demands urgent hospital treatment.

Surgical Treatment of Epilepsy

If the causative lesion is, for example, a benign tumour, surgical removal may be possible and would offer a high chance of cure although epileptic attacks may still recur due to residual brain damage. If the E.E.G. repeatedly shows a focal origin in an area of the brain which can be excised, for example, the anterior part of one frontal or temporal lobe, neurosurgical treatment can be undertaken even when special X-ray investigations have failed to reveal a lesion.

Removal of the anterior 5–6 cms of the temporal lobe, sparing the superior temporal gyrus, is called *temporal lobectomy*. Such operations are suitable for only a small proportion of epileptics whose attacks prove resistant to medical treatment. Pathological examination of the removed tissue sometimes shows sclerosis or atrophy (shrinkage) with gliosis which is considered to be due to hypoxia resulting from birth trauma or status epilepticus in infancy.

CHAPTER 11

TUMOURS

Pathology

Tumours are abnormal growths (neoplasms) and are classified as primary or secondary. A primary tumour consists of microscopic cells that are similar to those of the tissues in which it develops. These cells proliferate and the resulting tumour may be benign or malignant.

A *benign* tumour grows slowly, and does not infiltrate or invade locally or spread to other parts of the body. It thus remains confined to the structure of origin, is often encapsulated and its main effects are due to compression of surrounding tissues.

A *malignant* tumour infiltrates the tissues in which it develops and invades neighbouring structures; many malignant tumours metastasise, i.e. spread to other parts of the body, the malignant cells of the primary growth infiltrating into the lymphatic or blood circulation and so are transported to organs elsewhere. These cells then form secondary tumours or deposits (metastases) which continue to grow and spread in the same way. Secondary tumours are thus the result of the metastasis of primary malignant tumours and consist of cells similar to those of the primary tumour.

Tumour cells as seen under a microscope have characteristic shapes and patterns resembling the cells of the tissues from which they arise. The most malignant tumours consist of mainly primitive and poorly differentiated cells which tend to proliferate rapidly. Cell multiplication is the result of mitosis and the demonstration of mitotic cells under the microscope usually indicates that the tumour is malignant.

The names given to tumours (whether benign or malignant) frequently end in the suffix '-oma', e.g. meningioma, astrocytoma —the first part of the name indicating the structure or type of cells from which the tumour originates. The suffix '-blastoma' implies that the tumour is composed of blast or primitive cells which are usually highly malignant. Some malignant tumours are referred to as carcinoma (e.g. of bronchus or breast) and these are amongst the commonest forms of cancer.

INTRACRANIAL TUMOURS

Primary intracranial tumours originate from the structures within the skull, e.g. the meninges (*meningioma*) or within the brain (e.g. *glioma*). The secondary intracranial tumours (metastases) originate from a primary growth elsewhere in the body, usually a carcinoma of the lung or breast.

With any intracranial tumour, the clinical effects are due to:

(1) local symptoms and signs,
(2) epilepsy, focal or generalised, and
(3) raised intracranial pressure.

These may occur singly or in combination.

Meningioma

This is a primary tumour of the meninges and can develop in the spinal canal as well as intracranially; it is commoner in women.

Meningiomas are benign tumours, i.e. they grow relatively slowly, do not actively infiltrate the brain and do not metastasise. The local effects are due to direct compression or displacement of the brain in which they may become deeply embedded. Raised intracranial pressure eventually develops and, if not relieved, death will ensue. These tumours usually grow into spherical shaped or irregular, lobulated masses with a relatively small point of attachment where the tumour originated from the dura, but sometimes they extend as a solid layer (meningioma en plaque). They may also produce thickening of the overlying bone (hyperostosis) and occasionally erode through the skull to form a palpable or visible swelling on the head. There is a predilection for certain sites so that the symptoms and signs will vary with the structures involved.

(1) *Olfactory groove* meningioma will compress or displace the olfactory nerve and cause loss of the sense of smell (anosmia). As it increases in size it may press on the optic nerve causing loss of

vision with primary optic atrophy. Raised intracranial pressure may supervene with generalised headache, vomiting and papilloedema. Olfactory groove meningiomas also compress the frontal lobes of the cerebral hemispheres causing changes in personality, behaviour and mood, often with disinhibition and mental and intellectual deterioration. Tumours in this situation can present with various types of epilepsy including status epilepticus.

If the frontal lobe of the dominant cerebral hemisphere is involved and the tumour impinges on the speech area, this will cause dysphasia. A monoparesis or hemiplegia eventually develops with a grasp reflex, i.e. the hand grasps involuntarily or reflexly anything that touches the palm. This is a primitive reflex seen normally during the first few months of life in infants, who grasp a finger or other object placed across the palm and do not let go unless forced to do so. Another manifestation of frontal lobe lesions is loss of control of micturition, usually with incontinence.

(2) *Parasagittal* or *convexity* meningioma originates from the falx near the sagittal sinus or the dura mater over the convexity of the cerebral hemispheres. Parasagittal meningioma may present with focal epilepsy starting in the opposite foot with transient motor or sensory disturbances which later become persistent and progressive.

(3) *Sphenoidal ridge* meningioma arises from the region of the greater or lesser wing of the sphenoid bone. The tumour enlarges in the middle fossa to compress the temporal lobe causing temporal lobe epilepsy (see Chapter 10). If the tumour is on the side of the dominant cerebral hemisphere, dysphasia develops. Involvement of the lower fibres of the optic radiation will produce contralateral homonymous upper quadrantic visual field defects, progressing to a complete homonymous hemianopia if the whole of the optic radiation becomes involved.

(4) *Parasellar* meningioma occurs around the pituitary fossa. The tumour presses on the optic nerves, chiasm or tracts, causing the corresponding visual field defects and primary optic atrophy.

(5) *Tentorial* meningioma arises from the tentorium cerebelli and grows either in a supra-tentorial direction compressing one or both cerebral hemispheres, or downwards (infra-tentorially) into the posterior fossa compressing the cerebellum or brain stem. In the latter case there will be signs of cerebellar dysfunction, which may include dysarthria (see Chapter 7).

The diagnosis of a meningioma may sometimes be suspected if

the plain X-rays of the skull show a localised area of erosion or sclerosis of the bone overlying the tumour. Arteriography may show displacement of vessels by the tumour, which typically shows a 'radiological blush' due to its vascularity (the blush resulting from filling of the tumour blood vessels with the radiopaque dye).

Many meningiomas can be completely removed and the prognosis is usually good. There is relief of the raised intracranial pressure, the focal neurological signs regress and may clear completely if the damage has not been too severe or long standing. Epileptic attacks also cease unless there has been irreversible damage of the cerebral cortex by the tumour prior to removal. Because the tumour may have interfered with the blood supply to part of the brain, neurological disability may prove to be permanent. It is not always possible to remove the tumour completely so that, some time after operation, the signs recur due to regrowth of the remaining tumour. This occasionally takes on a more rapidly growing form with less differentiated cells (meningiosarcoma). Because of the danger of recurrence, radiotherapy may be advised postoperatively.

Dysphasia results from a meningioma pressing on the speech area, and dysarthria from a posterior fossa meningioma involving the brain stem or cerebellum; these speech disorders, like the other effects, will be progressive unless the tumour is removed. Post-operative speech therapy is indicated to enhance recovery of language function and compensate for residual defects. Various factors influence the prognosis for recovery of speech (see Chapter 5).

Glioma

Gliomas are more common than meningiomas. Gliomas are primary malignant tumours of the brain originating from the glial cells, i.e. astrocytes, oligodendrocytes and microglia which form the connective tissue of the brain. These tumours are named according to the microscopic appearances of the cells.

The commonest type of glioma is an *astrocytoma* which is derived from cells of the astrocyte type. These tumours are locally malignant and infiltrate brain substance but do not metastasise outside the nervous system. The rate of growth and spread of astrocytomas vary and different grades of malignancy can be recognised microscopically. These grades are numbered 1–4, the most malignant being grade 4 (glioblastoma multiforme or spongioblastoma) which is recognised by the presence of undifferentiated primitive cells frequently seen in mitosis. Tumours of this type often present with epilepsy, symptoms and signs of raised intracranial pressure, and focal neurological deficits. There is progessive deterioration leading to death often within a few months from the onset of symptoms. Grade 1 astrocytoma can be very slowly growing, the first indication of a cerebral lesion (e.g. a focal fit) occurring sometimes as long as 5, 10 or even 15 years before death.

Oligodendrogliomas are derived from the oligodendrocytes, and as they are usually very slowly growing, calcification often occurs in them and can be seen radiologically.

The prognosis with gliomas is usually poor since infiltration of the brain substance prevents removal of all of the tumour, which probably extends further than is obvious to the naked eye at operation. Complete removal and cure is occasionally achieved e.g. if an astrocytoma grade 1 is diagnosed early and removed in toto by temporal lobectomy. Sometimes, large cysts form within an astrocytoma, fill up with fluid and cause raised intracranial pressure. These can be aspirated with relief of pressure symptoms. The more malignant gliomas form many abnormal blood vessels so that the tumour is very vascular. Haemorrhages are then liable to occur spontaneously or on attempted biopsy (i.e. surgical removal of a small piece of tumour for diagnostic microscopic examination). Although radiotherapy is given in some cases, the results are not very encouraging as these tumours are rarely radiosensitive.

Other cerebral tumours

Ependymoma are derived from the cells lining the ventricles These tumours are derived from the cells lining the ventricles (ependyma) and are situated deeply in the substance of the brain. They are not common, nor are the other tumours which develop in the cerebral hemispheres e.g. colloid cysts of the third ventricle, cholesteatoma, papillomas of the choroid plexus and pinealoma.

The pineal gland is situated in the posterior wall of the 3rd ventricle in the midline. A *pinealoma* is a tumour of this gland and may extend forwards to block the flow of C.S.F. so causing obstructive hydrocephalus (see Chapter 14). Other effects are variable, depending upon the main directions of growth. There may be compression or invasion of the cerebral hemispheres or the tumours may extend downwards compressing the posterior aspect of the mid-brain at the level of the corpora quadrigemina. This interferes with conjugate eye movements, typically causing defective upward gaze.

Pinealomas as a rule are not accessible for neurosurgical removal, but radiotherapy is effective in some. The hydrocephalus can be treated surgically, by making a shunt so that the C.S.F. can by-pass the obstruction and be absorbed. The most popular procedure now is to insert a Spitz-Holter valve; this is connected with a tube put into the lateral ventricle and a pumping device takes the C.S.F. into the jugular vein in the neck.

Pituitary tumours

The pituitary gland (often called the conductor of the endocrine orchestra because it secretes hormones which govern other ductless glands) is situated at the base of the brain. Several types of tumour, depending on the main type of cell, may develop. The commonest are pituitary *adenomas* which are most frequently chromophobe, but eosinophil and basophil types also occur. *Craniopharyngioma* (i.e. tumours developing from embryonic remnants near the pituitary) are less common.

The main clinical effects of pituitary tumours are:

1. *Endocrine*

(a) Hypopituitarism—due to compression of the pituitary gland by the tumour interfering with production of one or more pituitary hormones, so causing secondary defects of gonadal (sex), adrenal or thyroid functions.

(b) acromegaly—due to excessive production of growth hormone by the tumour cells.

(c) Cushing's syndrome—due to excessive production of adrenocorticotrophic hormone (A.C.T.H.) by the tumour cells.

2. *Compression of optic pathways*

The optic chiasm lies anterior to and above the pituitary fossa and is particularly vulnerable to pressure from an expanding pituitary tumour. The characteristic visual field defect which results from chiasmal compression is bitemporal hemianopia (see

Fig. 7) due to damage to the nasal crossing fibres of the optic nerve which convey images from the temporal halves of both visual fields. Neurosurgical treatment is indicated for relief of failing vision.

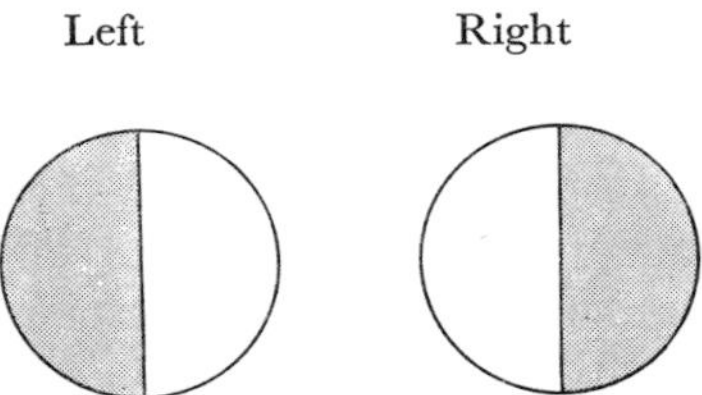

FIG. 7. Bitemporal hemianopia.

3. *The effects of suprasellar extension*
Pituitary tumours can grow upwards out of the sella turcica and extend into the anterior or middle fossae. This will compress the adjacent temporal or frontal areas of the cerebral hemispheres, causing focal epilepsy (e.g. with temporal lobe features) or motor deficits (e.g. facial weakness of U.M.N. type). Dysphasia is a rare complication as the speech area lies on the lateral surface of the dominant cerebral hemisphere.

CEREBELLAR TUMOURS

The main *primary* cerebellar tumours are:

(1) astrocytoma
(2) haemangioblastoma
(3) medulloblastoma

Astrocytoma of the cerebellum

In children astrocytomas occur more frequently in the cerebellum than in the cerebral hemisphere. They are often cystic, slowly progressive and invade the cerebellum and brain stem. Occasionally they originate in and remain confined to the brain stem.

Haemangioblastoma

These are usually benign encapsulated tumours, composed mainly of blood vessel-forming cells. Often cystic, they may contain large amounts of fluid with a relatively small tumour embedded in the wall (mural nodule). These tumours can often be removed completely.

Medulloblastoma

These occur almost invariably in children and are very malignant tumours of the brain stem and cerebellar vermis. They are locally invasive and extend deeply into the floor of the fourth ventricle. Being friable, fragments break off and circulate in the C.S.F., becoming attached to the surface of other parts of the neuraxis, e.g. the spinal cord. This type of spread is called 'seeding'. Medulloblastomas are initially radiosensitive but nearly always recur so that the prognosis is poor.

METASTASES

Secondary tumours (metastases) in the cerebellum are not infrequent, the commonest site of the primary tumour being the lung or breast.

ACOUSTIC NEUROMA

A neuroma or neurofibroma is a benign primary tumour which may grow from the sheath of any (cranial or spinal) nerve. The commonest cranial nerve to be affected is the 8th cranial (acoustic) nerve. Very rarely there may be bilateral acoustic neuromas. In a small percentage of cases (10–15%) an acoustic neuroma may be associated with multiple neurofibromatosis (Von Recklinghausen's disease). In this condition, the tumours grow on the peripheral nerves in the skin and subcutaneous tissue; it is often associated with pigmented (café-au-lait) patches on the skin. Skeletal deformities can develop and tumours on the spinal nerve roots may compress the spinal cord.

An acoustic neuroma interferes with 8th nerve functions (auditory and vestibular) causing unilateral deafness, tinnitus and vertigo. The deafness is perceptive in type and progressive. Tinnitus in the hallucination of sound and the patient may be aware, for example, of a continuous hum in the affected ear. Vertigo is the hallucination of movement, usually rotatory, similar to the sensation experienced immediately after getting off a roundabout.

Situated in the cerebello-pontine angle, an acoustic neuroma will also cause the following:

(1) involvement of other cranial nerves, particularly the 7th and 5th, resulting in facial weakness and numbness, including loss of the corneal reflex.

(2) compression of the cerebellar hemisphere with inco-ordination of the arm and leg on the same side, nystagmus and dysarthria.

(3) compression of the brain stem producing pyramidal (U.M.N.) signs.

(4) raised intracranial pressure—viz, headache, vomiting and papilloedema.

As the tumour is benign and encapsulated, removal is usually possible but owing to its situation there may be technical difficulties. Since an expanding tumour will eventually prove fatal from increase in intracranial pressure or compression of the brain stem, neurosurgery is advisable and, when the tumour is small, results are satisfactory. Unfortunately the 7th cranial nerve, being in such close proximity to the 8th nerve during its course from the brain stem to the facial canal, is frequently compressed by the tumour and may have to be sacrificed during removal of the tumour. The facial palsy which ensues is disfiguring and initially may cause dysarthria; patients usually learn to compensate for this and pronounce words quite clearly by talking out of the unaffected side of the mouth. Plastic surgery can improve the cosmetic effect and facio-hypoglossal nerve anastomosis provides reasonable function in the facial muscles, the unilateral paralysis and wasting of the tongue (resulting from division of the hypoglossal nerve) being relatively unimportant.

The dysarthria resulting from damage to the cerebellum or the lower cranial nerves often persists post-operatively and speech therapy is indicated to improve articulation. With involvement of the 10th cranial (vagus) nerve, nasal voice and dysphonia may occur but usually improve post-operatively.

CHAPTER 12

VASCULAR DISORDERS

Blood Supply of the Brain

Four arteries in the neck carry the blood supply to the brain, namely the internal carotid and vertebral arteries on each side.

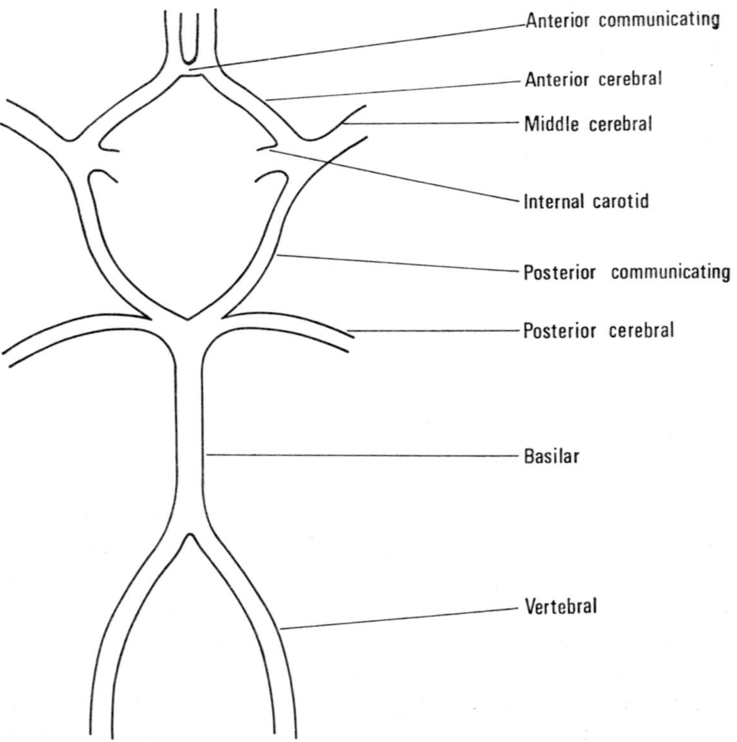

FIG. 8. Diagram of the Circle of Willis. (From *The Management of Cerebro-vascular Disease*, by J. Marshall, 2nd Ed. Churchill, London, 1968).

The internal carotid arteries pass through the foramen lacerum at the base of the skull to follow a tortuous intracranial course (the carotid syphon). Above this each gives off the ophthalmic artery and then terminates by dividing into anterior and middle cerebral arteries. The vertebral arteries pass up through the vertebral canals in the transverse processes of the cervical vertebrae, coil around the arch of the atlas on each side and pass through the foramen magnum, above which they join to form the basilar artery; this artery ascends in the midline along the anterior aspect of the brain stem to which it gives off paired branches. At the upper level of the mid-brain the basilar artery terminates by dividing into the two posterior cerebral arteries. *The Circle of Willis* (see Fig. 8) is completed by the posterior communicating arteries, which join the posterior cerebral to the internal carotid arteries and by the anterior communicating artery which joins the right and left anterior cerebral arteries.

STROKES

A stroke is a catastrophic or potentially serious disorder of brain function due to interference with the circulation. The three main causes are:

1. haemorrhage,
2. infarction,
3. transient ischaemic attacks ('litte strokes').

1. HAEMORRHAGE

Haemorrhage results from rupture of the wall of a blood vessel so that blood escapes from the circulation, either into the subarachnoid space (subarachnoid haemorrhage), the substance of the brain (intracerebral or intracerebellar) or into the ventricle (intraventricular); the blood may clot forming a haematoma.

Intracranial haemorrhage usually causes sudden headache, often with loss of consciousness. Within a few minutes, there are usually signs of meningeal irritation due to blood in the subarachnoid space, e.g. photophobia (dislike of light) and neck stiffness, which disappear if coma supervenes.

The commonest causes of intracranial haemorrhage are:

(1) Atheroma and Arteriosclerosis, with hypertension,
(2) Aneurysm and Angioma,
(3) Bleeding Diseases,
(4) Trauma.

Atheroma and Arteriosclerosis

The three layers of a vessel wall are (1) the *intima* which is the inner endothelial lining, (2) the *media* or muscular and elastic layer, and (3) the *adventitia* which is the connective tissue surrounding the blood vessel. Atheroma is the name given to the change in the arteries due to deposition of plaques of cholesterol in the intima. It usually affects the smaller and medium sized arteries and causes narrowing of the lumen. Arteriosclerosis occurs when the elastic tissue degenerates, the wall of the artery becomes thickened, irregular and tortuous, and micro-aneurysms may form on the capillaries. High blood pressure (which is commonly associated with degenerative arterial disease) will further aggravate the liability of the vessel wall to rupture, resulting in haemorrhage.

Aneurysm

This is a dilation of the artery, usually at a point of bifurcation, due to congenital weakness in the media. Most aneurysms are found on the main arteries of the circle of Willis, approximately 30% arising from the anterior group (i.e. the anterior cerebral and anterior communicating arteries), 30% directly from the internal carotid artery, usually at the level of the junction with the posterior communicating artery and 30% from the middle cerebral arteries. The remaining 10% are situated on the various other intracranial arteries, i.e. vertebral and basilar or their branches, or on the peripheral branches of the cerebral arteries.

The wall of an aneurysm is more liable to rupture as the patient gets older, when atheromatous changes become superimposed and hypertension develops. The seriousness of rupture of an intracranial aneurysm is evidenced by the fact that about

50% of patients die within four weeks and few survive more than 2 or 3 haemorrhages.

Another complication occurs if the sac of the aneurysm enlarges and compresses the neighbouring structures; for example, compression of the third cranial (oculo-motor) nerve by an aneurysm of the internal carotid artery at its junction with the posterior communicating artery causes an oculo-motor palsy, viz. ptosis, dilated pupil and paralysis of the external ocular muscles (excluding the superior oblique and lateral rectus muscles).

Angioma

An angioma is a congenital malformation consisting of a mass of abnormal blood vessels. It may be situated within the substance of one cerebral hemisphere or the brain stem, or superficially on the surface, sometimes extending deeply into the cerebral hemisphere in the shape of a wedge. The size varies from minute angiomas visible only with a microscope to extremely large ones involving almost the whole of one hemisphere; they are supplied by some or all of the main arteries of the circle of Willis. Instead of blood taking its normal time and course through the capillaries of the brain, these congenital anomalies form large arterio-venous communications or shunts which tend to deprive the underlying area of the brain of its normal blood supply. The vessels making up the angioma are abnormally thin and liable to rupture so that subarachnoid or intracerebral haemorrhages are common complications. Rupture of an angioma tends to occur at an earlier age than with an aneurysm and is less commonly fatal so that there may be a history of several haemorrhages.

Other complications of angioma are epilepsy and persistent neurological deficits such as dysphasia, depending on which part of the brain is involved.

Bleeding Diseases

Subarachnoid and intracerebral haemorrhages, often minute but multiple, can result from haemorrhagic diseases in which there is some general disorder of the clotting mechanism of the blood, e.g. when there is a deficiency of platelets as in thrombocytopenia and some cases of leukaemia. Intracranial haemorrhage may also occur as a complication of anticoagulant therapy.

Trauma

Head injuries may cause haemorrhage or contusion in the substance of the brain, sometimes with bleeding into the subarachnoid space (traumatic subarachnoid haemorrhage). Bleeding may also occur into the extradural or subdural spaces forming localised clots (extradural or subdural haematoma); the resultant rise in intracranial pressure can cause severe, even fatal, complications because of compression and distortion of the cerebral hemispheres or brain stem. In any severe head injury with intracranial haemorrhage there may be a fracture of the skull and concussion. Concussion is the 'knock-out' of brain function that follows a head injury, i.e. the immediate loss of consciousness, confusion and amnesia that are reversible and not due to any *visible* brain damage which may or may not coexist.

Investigations

Lumbar puncture in sub-arachnoid haemorrhage reveals uniformly blood-stained C.S.F. instead of the normally clear and colourless fluid. If the specimen is centrifuged or allowed to stand, the supernatant fluid has a yellow tinge (*xanthochromia*).

X-rays of the skull may show a fracture, or displacement of the calcified pineal gland, for example, by an intracranial haematoma. (The pineal gland appears calcified in the skull X-rays of about 50% of normal people and should be in the midline). Echo-encephalography (using an ultrasonoscope) may also indicate shift of midline structures and scanning techniques using radioactive isotopes may demonstrate the lesion.

The most important diagnostic test is arteriography, a radiological technique involving the injection of a radio-opaque dye into either of the carotid or vertebral arteries in the neck. Following injection the dye is carried with the circulating blood into the intracranial blood vessels which are then revealed by X-rays. An intracranial haematoma (extradural, subdural or intracerebral) is demonstrated by displacement of the blood vessels; for example, instead of the anterior cerebral artery lying almost in the midline, it may be displaced towards the opposite side; an aneurysm is shown as a small diverticulum on an artery; an angioma as a tangle of knotted vessels on the surface of, and perhaps extending deeply into, one cerebral hemisphere;

atheroma and arteriosclerosis are revealed by narrowing, irregularity and tortuousity of the arteries.

Treatment

Intracranial haematoma can be removed surgically. If an aneurysm is found, the management depends on its exact situation since many are now accessible to surgery by ligation or clipping of the neck of the aneurysm close to its junction with the wall of the artery. This prevents any future rupture as the aneurysmal sac is excluded from the circulation. An alternative method is to wrap a piece of muscle or synthetic material around the fundus of the sac to strengthen the wall and prevent any recurrent rupture. Yet another method of treatment is to reduce the pressure in the arteries leading to the aneurysm by ligation of the common carotid artery in the neck. When the patient is hypertensive, the blood pressure can be effectively lowered by hypotensive drugs.

2. INFARCTION

Infarction is death of tissue (necrosis) due to impairment of the blood supply (ischaemia). If the cells of the nervous system (neurones) are deprived of their blood supply for more than a few minutes, they cannot survive and there will be an area of cerebral infarction. The extent of the infarct and the resultant neurological deficits will depend not only on which vessel is obstructed but also on the capacity of neighbouring arteries to supplement the deficient blood supply, i.e. develop a *collateral circulation*.

The two main causes of prolonged or severe ischaemia sufficient to produce infarction are (a) thrombosis and (b) embolism.

(a) Thrombosis

Intravascular clot formation (thrombosis) is commonly due to atheroma with slowing of the blood flow. The clot causing the obstruction may develop either in the intra- or extra-cranial parts of the carotid and vertebral arteries; this is liable to result in cerebral infarction particularly if the intracranial vessels are arteriosclerotic, which reduces the capacity to form a collateral circulation.

Investigations

The cerebro-spinal fluid is nearly always clear (i.e. not obviously blood-stained) and carotid arteriography may show the point of obstruction in the affected artery. At least 20% of strokes are due to occlusion of the extracranial part of the internal carotid artery in the neck just above the bifurcation of the common carotid artery.

Treatment

In some cases it may be possible to remove the thrombus surgically, if it is near the origin of the internal carotid artery in the neck and if the block is not complete. This may be justified if serious cerebral deficit has not already developed, but the long term results of such procedures are still uncertain.

Anti-coagulant therapy is contra-indicated in acute cerebral infarction due to thrombosis because of the danger of bleeding into the infarcted brain tissue. Severe hypertension can be treated with hypotensive drugs but care must be taken not to reduce the blood pressure below a certain level as this may further impair the cerebral circulation and interfere with recovery.

(b) Embolism

An embolus is a fragment of clot or other substance, e.g. fat, air, aggregations of platelets, fibrin or cholesterol, which is carried in the circulation from one part of the body and obstructs a blood vessel elsewhere. Embolism is liable to occur in various heart diseases, for example when the auricles are not contracting properly (auricular fibrillation) so that the blood in the auricles becomes stagnant and forms clots. Fragments break off, pass through the auricular-ventricular valves (mitral or tricuspid) to be expelled via the main arteries and carried in the circulation, eventually obstructing smaller blood vessels such as the cerebral arteries supplying the brain. If the obstruction is not relieved (for example by further fragmentation or absorption of the clot) and if the collateral circulation is inadequate, the area of brain involved will become infarcted. Embolism also occurs in myocardial disease secondary to coronary thrombosis, i.e. a clot in the coronary arteries supplying the heart, so that there is infarction of the heart muscle (myocardial infarction). This may involve the inner lining of the heart (endocardium) with formation of a clot on the endocardial surface. If this fragments, emboli may then be carried via the aorta into any of the main arteries in the body and cerebral embolism may result.

Cerebral embolism presents with an extremely sudden disturbance of function, the resulting signs depending upon which part of the brain is rendered ischaemic. Dysphasia and hemiplegia due to a cerebral embolus will have an acute onset followed by improvement. Although recovery in some cases is slow and incomplete, in others there is no loss of consciousness and the prognosis is excellent. Specific medical or surgical treatment is directed to the underlying cause of the clot formation and anti-coagulent therapy is used in some cases.

3. TRANSIENT ISCHAEMIC ATTACKS

Occlusion of blood vessels by thrombosis or embolism is not necessarily complete and the ischaemia may be insufficient to cause infarction. There are also other causes of transient ischaemia which may produce temporary or relatively minor disturbances of cerebral function, sometimes referred to as 'little strokes'.

Spasm of cerebral blood vessels (narrowing due to contraction of the muscle wall) is occasionally seen in arteriograms and at operation. Spasm is a temporary, reversible phenomenon which interferes with the blood supply and causes transient attacks of cerebral ischaemia. This results in focal cerebral symptoms and, if the period of ischaemia is short, infarction does not occur and recovery follows when the spasm clears and the blood supply is restored. Spasm or vasoconstriction producing cerebral or brain stem ischaemia in this way is thought to account for the transient premonitory symptoms (e.g. visual, sensory and sometimes speech disturbances etc.) which occur in *migraine*, the headache being associated with the subsequent vasodilatation.

Conditions causing fall in cardiac output and blood pressure also produce transient cerebral ischaemia and this is the mechanism of fainting (*syncope*). The fall in blood pressure results in defective blood supply to the brain stem and cerebral hemispheres producing the symptoms of faintness, dizziness, blurred vision and nausea, etc., leading to loss of consciousness; the patient falls to the ground and this lowering of the head restores the blood supply to the brain so that recovery is rapid. There are many causes of syncope e.g. vaso-vagal attacks, cough syncope, hypotension and cardiac disorders such as heart block (*Stokes-Adams attacks*).

Transient ischaemic attacks affecting the cerebral hemispheres or brain stem are commonly encountered in arteriosclerotic patients with narrowing (stenosis) of the internal carotid or vertebral arteries. If this can be confirmed by arteriography and if the narrowed segment is localised in an accessible situation in a relatively young patient, it may be treated surgically so removing the obstruction to the blood supply.

The vertebral arteries are vulnerable to obstruction in the vertebral canal of the cervical spine and in their upper part as they curve round the transverse processes of the atlas. Excessive or prolonged movements of the head and neck can interfere with the circulation via the vertebral arteries, particularly when these are arteriosclerotic. In middle aged and elderly subjects, there is often cervical spondylosis, i.e. degeneration of the cervical spine with narrowing of the disc spaces, the small joints becoming deformed with bony irregularities (osteophytes). These may impinge on the vertebral arteries and impede the circulation especially when the head is turned or the neck extended.

Transient ischaemic attacks affecting the brain stem are referred to as 'vertebro-basilar insufficiency'. The symptoms are due to the disturbances of brain stem function resulting from involvement of cranial nerve nuclei, e.g. defects of eye movements and diplopia (3rd, 4th and 6th), sensory loss on the face (5th), facial weakness (7th), tinnitus, deafness, vertigo and nystagmus (8th), loss of palatal sensation (9th), palatal weakness, dysphagia, dysphonia and dysarthria (10th, 11th and 12th). Involvement of the sympathetic fibres in the brain stem will cause Horner's syndrome (partial ptosis, constriction of the pupil, enophthalmos and loss of sweating on the forehead of the affected side). In addition there may be inco-ordination and ataxia of the limbs, nystagmus and ataxic dysarthria from ischaemia of the cerebellum and its connections.

As mentioned previously, if the ischaemia is prolonged beyond the critical period, infarction will result and the same neurological deficits may become permanent. Transient ischaemic episodes may recur repeatedly and herald the onset of a major stroke. Sometimes it is possible to relieve these transient attacks, for example by restriction of neck movements (using a collar), anti-coagulant therapy or drugs which improve the circulation so increasing the flow of blood through the narrowed vessels; a major stroke may occasionally be averted in this way.

CHAPTER 13

INFECTIONS

Infections are the result of invasion of the body by micro-organisms such as bacteria and viruses. These organisms vary in virulence, i.e. their capacity to spread and cause disease.

The factors which determine the result of an infection are the resistance or susceptibility of the host tissues (a high standard of general health and well-being will tend to improve resistance to infection), the virulence of the infecting organism and the sensitivity of the organism to treatment.

Bacteria are microscopic organisms which are universally disseminated. Each organism consists of one cell which has the capacity to multiply but only some produce disease (i.e. are pathogenic). Bacteria have various shapes, e.g. round (cocci), rod shaped (bacilli), but a high-power microscope is necessary to see these.

Viruses are also unicellular organisms but are smaller than bacteria. Infections due to viruses include the common cold, influenza, measles, poliomyelitis, small pox and chicken pox, herpes simplex and zoster. Viruses may infect the nervous system and cause meningitis or encephalitis (inflammation of the meninges or brain). Encephalitis may be diffuse and involve large areas of the brain, or localised and result in abscess formation.

Inflammation

Tissues which become infected with an organism produce an inflammatory reaction i.e. there is redness and swelling due to increase of the local blood supply (vaso-dilatation) with seepage of fluid and white blood cells (leucocytes and macrophages). Necrosis in the centre of the inflamed area leads to pus formation and a surrounding capsule is formed by fibrous tissue. The pus-filled cavity increases in size and at the point of least resistance comes to the surface, where it may burst spontaneously, or require surgical evacuation of the pus. Provided that the infection is overcome by virtue of the resistance of the tissues and treatment with appropriate antibiotics, the inflammatory reaction will subside.

Abscess

An abscess is a localised pocket of infection containing pus, e.g. a boil is an abscess in the skin. In some parts of the body, if the pus cannot be evacuated, the abscess increases in size and penetrates deeply to cause increasing damage by compression.

A cerebral abscess is the result of an infection which reaches the brain either by direct spread from the middle ear (otitis media), or sinuses (sinusitis), or via the blood stream e.g. from the lungs (pneumonia or pulmonary abscess). The cerebral abscess acts as an intracranial space-occupying lesion producing symptoms and signs of raised intracranial pressure, viz. headache, vomiting and papilloedema. Local effects are determined by its situation e.g. it may cause focal epilepsy or neurological signs, including dysphasia if the speech area is involved.

Otitis media and mastoiditis

Infection of the middle ear may penetrate the petrous bone spreading anteriorly into the middle cranial fossa to involve the temporal lobe, or posteriorly into the posterior fossa to involve the adjacent cerebellar hemisphere. Abscesses can form in other parts of the brain, even on the side opposite to the infected ear, and may be multiple, indicating that the spread has been via the blood stream.

Local meningeal reaction or rupture of an intracerebral abscess leads to meningitis. Other complications from otitis media include lateral sinus thrombosis and cortical thrombo-phlebitis.

The organisms that cause these infections are most commonly the staphylococcus, Bacterium coli, Haemophilus influenzae and Proteus.

Meningitis

Inflammation of the meninges usually results from spread of a local infection or is a complication of a systemic infection, frequently viral. Bacterial meningitis in adults may be due to the meningococcus or pneumococcus and in children to Haemophilus influenzae, although any of the bacteria already mentioned may be responsible. Meningococcal meningitis (cerebro-spinal or 'spotted fever') occurs in epidemic form and, before the discovery of sulphonamides and antibiotics, was often fatal, but nowadays it is more amenable to treatment. It was called 'spotted-fever' because in fulminating cases, purpura (minute haemorrhagic spots) developed in the skin. Haemorrhage occasionally occurred in the adrenal glands causing death from adrenal failure.

Many of the complications of meningitis are the result of inflammatory exudate forming mainly at the base of the brain, so damaging the cranial nerves. Involvement of the 8th cranial (auditory) nerves, causing deafness, is most frequent, but damage to this nerve can also result from the toxic effects of streptomycin (one of the antibiotics used in the treatment of tuberculosis).

Tuberculosis

Infection with the tubercle bacillus (T.B.) most commonly involves the lungs (pulmonary tuberculosis). All forms of tuberculosis including tuberculous meningitis are now relatively rare in England but still common in Asia. Tuberculous abscesses more often occur in the cerebellar than cerebral hemispheres and are complications of tuberculosis of tissues elsewhere (e.g. the lungs), the infecting organisms (tubercle bacilli) being carried to the brain via the blood stream. As the tuberculous abscess enlarges, raised intracranial pressure develops. Alternatively, a chronic granuloma (tuberculoma) is formed and may exist in the brain for months or even years without causing symptoms. It may become inactive and calcified showing up on plain X-rays of the skull as a rounded irregular calcified mass.

Syphilis

This is one of the venereal diseases which may produce local genital symptoms when contracted, and then remain latent to produce manifestations of involvement of the nervous system (neurosyphilis) many years later. There is also a congenital form of the disease due to transmission to the foetus by an infected mother. The spirochaete which causes syphilis, Treponema pallidum, is a cork-screw shaped micro-organism, which invades the tissues to cause the specific inflammatory reaction of the disease.

Neurosyphilis is now relatively rare, but the classical types are still recognised.

General paralysis of the insane (*G.P.I.*)

G.P.I. develops after a latent period following the acute infection, sometimes as long as 10–20 years later. The disease affects the cerebral hemispheres causing generalised atrophy, particularly of the cortex. The mental, intellectual and personality deterioration (dementia) is progressive unless early treatment with penicillin is given. There are generalised tremors, involving particularly the hands, lips and tongue. The tremor of the hands is usually fine and rapid, but the tremor of the tongue is sometimes coarse with backwards and forwards movements, aptly described as 'trombone tremor'. Bilateral pyramidal signs with increased reflexes, clonus and extensor plantar responses are often present. There is a characteristic type of dysarthria which may be due to a combination of factors, viz. the tremor of the tongue, pseudobulbar palsy (due to bilateral upper motor neurone involvement), and cortical atrophy affecting the motor part of the speech area.

In all forms of neurosyphilis, pupillary abnormalities are frequently seen. The most characteristic is the *Argyll Robertson pupil*, which is small and irregular in outline; it does not react to light but does to accommodation. (Argyll Robertson was an Edinburgh ophthalmologist who first described these abnormalities).

Tabes dorsalis

The clinical picture is due to involvement of the posterior horns of the spinal cord, the posterior root ganglia of the spinal nerves and the sensory components of the cranial nerves. The main effects of tabes, therefore, are on the sensory system, depending upon the distribution of the segments affected. Involvement of the posterior nerve roots and ganglia often results in severe pain which is typically shooting or lancinating in character (lightning pains) causing sudden horizontally or vertically directed stabs, usually affecting the legs. Various visceral crises with bouts of severe pain may involve, for example, the bladder, stomach or larynx.

Loss of sensation occurs in various parts of the body, particularly the legs, ulnar aspects of the forearms and hands, over the chest and on the face and nose. Loss of superficial pain sensation is tested with a pin and, instead of the pinprick, the patient feels only a blunt touch. There is loss of deep pain sensation which is tested by squeezing the muscles and tendons (e.g. the tendo-Achilles) which are normally pain-sensitive. Loss of temperature sensation results in inability to differentiate between hot and cold and patients may sustain burns without feeling pain. The sensory fibres conveying pain and temperature sensations cross to the opposite side of the spinal cord and ascend in the lateral spino-thalamic tracts. The posterior roots also convey the senses of position and vibration, which are conveyed up the spinal cord by the fibres of the posterior columns. Because these are affected in patients with tabes dorsalis (the name literally means wasting of the dorsal columns), there is loss of position and vibration sense in the limbs. The position of various parts of the body can be checked visually, so the patient can compensate for loss of the sense of position, but there will be unsteadiness with a tendency to fall in the dark or with the eyes closed, e.g. when washing the face. Loss of position sense can be tested by asking the patient to stand up straight with the feet together; with the eyes open, balance is maintained but on closing the eyes, the patient sways and may fall due to loss of position sense in the feet and legs (Romberg's sign).

Because of interference with sensation to the skin, trophic changes may occur leading to ulceration which is often indolent and chronic. Interference with the sensation of joints leads to a painless form of arthropathy with gross deformities (Charcot's joints).

As a result of the loss of sensation from the bladder the patient may fail to appreciate when the bladder is full so that there is retention of urine, or overflow incontinence with an atonic bladder.

The loss of sensation also interferes with the reflex arc, so that the tendon reflexes in the limbs are reduced or absent.

Speech is not as a rule affected in tabes, except in cases having combined features of both tabes and G.P.I., which is then called *taboparesis*.

Meningo-vascular syphilis

As the name implies, the blood vessels and meninges are particularly involved. The meninges become inflamed and thickened due to a low grade meningitis in which headache is a marked feature. Thickening of the meninges at the base of the brain can also cause cranial nerve palsies. The lumen of the blood vessels, particularly those penetrating the meninges and supplying the surfaces of the brain, becomes narrowed and obliterated. Local areas of ischaemia result and cause focal epilepsy and neurological signs; according to the part involved, so aphasia, monoplegia or hemiplegia, homonymous hemianopia or hemianaesthesia may develop.

Gumma

This is a mass of granulomatous tissue due to syphilis and can occur in almost any part of the body, including the brain. An intracerebral gumma is exceedingly rare but acts as a space-occupying lesion causing raised intracranial pressure with focal neurological deficits depending upon its situation.

The *differential diagnosis* of neurosyphilis includes many disorders of the nervous system which it can resemble. Fortunately laboratory tests of the serum and C.S.F. are of great diagnostic value. Of these, the Wassermann Reaction (W.R.) is widely used, and is positive both in the serum and C.S.F. in most patients with active neurosyphilis. More refined tests have now been developed, including the treponemal immobilisation test (T.P.I). In some cases the W.R. becomes negative after treatment with penicillin, but the T.P.I. usually remains positive and so gives additional evidence of previous spirochaetal infection.

All forms of neurosyphilis are now rare, as the acute veneral infection can be effectively treated with penicillin and other antibiotics. Penicillin is the best prophylactic and curative treatment of neurosyphilis, and previous methods using malaria, arsenic and bismuth preparations have been superseded.

Poliomyelitis

This is an infection of the anterior horn cells and motor nuclei of the cranial nerves by the poliomyelitis virus. The acute stage lasts a few days with symptoms of a systemic illness, meningitis and sometimes encephalitis. If enough anterior horn cells in the spinal cord are involved paralysis of the lower motor neurone type occurs, typically in a patchy distribution and, if the motor nuclei in the brain stem are affected, bulbar palsy occurs with dysarthria, dysphonia and dysphagia (see Chapter 6).

Bulbar palsy and respiratory paralysis may necessitate artificial respiration, either with a tank type of respirator or tracheostomy with a pump respirator (intermittent positive pressure respirator—I.P.P.R.). Not all cases develop paralysis but, in those that do, recovery can take place provided that sufficient anterior horn cells or motor nuclei remain undamaged. Dead neurones cannot be replaced but probably more than half the number of functioning cells have to be damaged before any clinical weakness results. After the acute stage of the illness, further recovery of function is possible because certain muscles are capable of re-training and hypertrophy to compensate for those affected.

The serious epidemics that used to occur can be prevented by vaccination so that acute poliomyelitis is now a rarity.

CHAPTER 14

CONGENITAL MALFORMATIONS AND CEREBRAL PALSY

Congenital malformations are defined as abnormalities of structure present at birth. Infant mortality has decreased since the beginning of the century from 130 to nearly 20 per thousand live births; this progress is a reflection of improvements in ante-natal and obstetrical care together with advances in medical treatment of neonatal disorders. The number of children with congenital diseases has not changed so that they now provide a considerably higher proportion of neonatal mortality: whereas in 1900, 1/30 of the neonatal mortality was due to congenital abnormalities, now the proportion is approximately 1/4.

The incidence of congenital malformations depends on what is taken to be a malformation, whether still births are included and the age at which the incidence is assessed; approximately 1·5% at birth, it increases to 5% at one year of age. The C.N.S. is the commonest system affected by congenital malformation, 50% of all congenital lesions being neurological. Of 15 cases with congenital abnormalities, three will have spina-bifida, two anencephaly, two hydrocephalus, two heart disease, two cleft palate, and two mongolism, (the next commonest are club feet and dislocation of the hip): at least 7 of the 15 have C.N.S. involvement, or more if any of the cases of mongolism are mentally defective or retarded, as they often are. Other congenital conditions associated with mental defects include microcephaly and agenesis of the corpus callosum.

AETIOLOGY OF CONGENITAL MALFORMATIONS

The causes may be environmental or genetic.

A Environmental causes acting on the foetus via the mother include:

(1) dietary lack, either of protein, vitamin A, riboflavin, folic acid or thiamine.
(2) hormonal deficiency, e.g. of pituitary, thyroid or pancreas.
(3) chemical poisons, e.g. thalidomide, cortisone, antibiotics or nitrogen mustard.
(4) physical agents, e.g. radiation, hypoxia, hyperthermia.
(5) infections, e.g. rubella (german measles), toxoplasmosis, syphilis.

B Genetic causes include chromosome mutation which may affect many systems (e.g. mongolism) and gene mutation which usually affects only one system.

The type of congenital defect depends on the stage of development of the foetus when the damage occurs. Severe malformation of the C.N.S. such as anencephaly, hydrocephalus and spina bifida cystica occur in about 1/150 births.

Anencephaly is due to a defect of the closure of the embryological neural tube, the brain is virtually absent, and this is usually incompatible with life. It occurs in females more than males in the proportion of 5:1 and is often associated with an absence of the ganglion cells of the retina. There is a geographical variation in incidence, e.g. it is three times commoner in Ireland than in London.

Hydrocephalus is due to excessive accumulation of cerebro-spinal fluid (C.S.F.) within the cranial cavity and occurs in about 1/1000 births.

The C.S.F. is formed by the choroid plexuses, which consist of a mass of tangled capillaries and lie in the lateral, third and fourth ventricles. By a process of selective perfusion and filtration, the C.S.F. is produced from the plasma in the choroid plexuses, passes through the foramina in the roof of the fourth ventricle into the subarachnoid space, and is absorbed via the arachnoid villi into the dural venous sinuses.

Hydrocephalus is described as *obstructive* if the circulation of the C.S.F. is blocked in the third ventricle, aqueduct or fourth ventricle; an example is aqueduct stenosis (which can be inherited in a sex-linked recessive manner). The lateral ventricles dilate and the cerebral cortex becomes thin.

Communicating hydrocephalus occurs when the C.S.F. is not adequately absorbed from the subarachnoid space, which may be due to adhesions following meningitis.

The head circumference is normally 33.1 cm at birth, 36.8 cm at one month, 39.4 cm at two months and 46.8 cm at a year. A hydrocephalic head is abnormally large and globular in shape with protuberance of the forehead, bulging fontanelles and prominent scalp veins. There is a cracked-pot note on percussion of the skull. These are the effects of excessive C.S.F. under high pressure, occurring before the sutures of the baby's skull have fused. About 50% of cases arrest spontaneously and 25% reach adult life. The average I.Q. of hydrocephalics is 70, but 10% have an I.Q. above average. One third have no physical disability, but the others tend to have squints or various degrees of spasticity. Frequently there are other associated abnormalities present as well, e.g. an Arnold-Chiari malformation (i.e. prolongation of the cerebellar vermis and tonsils with lengthened medulla), or spina bifida cystica, and in these complicated cases the prognosis is worse.

Microcephaly (abnormal smallness of the head and brain) also occurs in approximately 1/1000 births; it is always associated with mental deficiency, and a third of the cases have epilepsy. Similar complications are associated with agenesis of the corpus callosum. The development of language functions are likely to be delayed, or will remain retarded and immature when there are severe mental and intellectual defects.

CEREBRAL PALSY

Cerebral palsy is not a disease entity but is the term used to cover a variety of neurological disorders which result from maldevelopment of, or damage to, the brain and present at the time of birth or early infancy. The abnormalities of brain function are reflected most obviously by defects of movement, failure of development of intellect, speech and language in the widest sense, and disturbances of behaviour and emotional control. In many of the children affected, the limbs are stiff and there are pyramidal signs; this is the group often referred to as 'spastics'. In 10% of cases, involuntary movements of an athetoid type—and not spasticity—constitute the principal disability while in about 5% of cases, the limbs are actually hypotonic and the child may be ataxic rather than spastic.

The incidence is approximately 7 per 100,000 births; of these one dies in infancy, two are mentally defective, one is severely handicapped, two can be rehabilitated, and one has only mild disability. It is the latter two groups that are most important from the point of view of speech therapy. Between 1 and 2 of every 1,000 school children have some form of cerebral palsy.

AETIOLOGY OF CEREBRAL PALSY

A. Pre-natal

1. Effect of maternal disorders on foetus in utero:
   - (a) anaemia or toxaemia of pregnancy.
   - (b) infections transmitted from mother, e.g. rubella, toxoplasmosis, syphilis.
   - (c) rhesus incompatibility.
2. Other embryological defects:
   - (a) agenesis
   - (b) porencephaly.

B. Peri-natal

1. prematurity.
2. birth trauma.
3. asphyxia, due to prolonged labour or difficult delivery.

C. Post-natal

1. infection, e.g. encephalitis.
2. cerebral venous thrombosis.

The proportion of children with cerebral palsy due to birth trauma has probably declined and more attention has been focussed on the possibility of agenesis or hypogenesis, i.e. a failure of development of part of the brain which occurs for reasons usually unknown. Anoxia during or shortly after delivery accounts for some cases.

Rubella (german measles) if contracted by the mother during the first three months of pregnancy, is particularly liable to cause congenital malformations.

During embryonic life, the primitive organs go through phases of rapid development at different times, during which they are vulnerable to infection. The stage of development of the foetus at the time of infection will determine which embryological structures are likely to sustain maximum damage and, presumably, the severity of virulence of the infection is also significant. The common congenital malformations which result from rubella are deafness, congenital heart disease, abnormalities of the eyes, and occasionally more serious defects such as anencephaly.

Rhesus incompatibility may cause serious defects of the foetus. This is dependent upon the mother being rhesus negative and forming antibodies which on mixing with the foetal circulation, interfere with the foetal red blood cells. This produces varying degrees of *erythroblastosis foetalis*. The effects range from anaemia to severe degrees of jaundice which may produce *kernicterus* where bile pigment is deposited in the basal ganglia, and sometimes more diffusely throughout the brain, causing the ganglionic athetoid type of cerebral palsy, often with mental deficiency and deafness. The level of maternal antibodies increases with succeeding pregnancies so that the degree of erythroblastosis increases with each baby born; two or more such pregnancies may result in a miscarriage or still-birth.

CLINICAL TYPES OF CEREBRAL PALSY

Although cerebral palsy usually reveals itself by a delay in development with failure to pass the intellectual and physical milestones at the appropriate age, most cases fall into a number of distinctive clinical syndromes.

(a) Spastic

This is the commonest variety of cerebral palsy with upper motor neurone signs affecting the limbs, e.g. spastic diplegia (Little's disease), monoplegia, hemiplegia or double hemiplegia; this may be associated with mental defect varying from slight mental retardation to amentia and many of these cases develop epilepsy.

The mildest cases show a delay of a few months in learning to walk with some clumsiness and unsteadiness of gait, symmetrical exaggeration of the lower limb reflexes and extensor plantar responses. Often the child is unable to walk until the 5th or 6th year and then does so with a characteristic 'scissors gait'; contractures tend to develop in the tendo-Achilles and posterior thigh muscles. In the most severe case, walking never becomes possible and all four limbs are spastic, indicating bilateral or diffuse involvement of cortico-spinal pathways.

If the left cerebral hemisphere is maldeveloped or damaged, the right hemisphere may become dominant, leading to 'pathological' left-handedness. Language function may develop normally, e.g. if taken over by the right cerebral hemisphere, but in some cases speech development is retarded and there may be specific language disorders (see Chapter 16). With diffuse bilateral cortical damage causing amentia, speech and language functions may fail to develop.

Dysarthria is either due to a localised cortical defect causing articulatory apraxia or more commonly to pseudo-bulbar palsy resulting from bilateral involvement of cortico-bulbar fibres.

(b) Athetoid

This is sometimes called the ganglionic or extrapyramidal type due to involvement of the basal ganglia or other parts of the extra-pyramidal system. It produces disorders of tone and posture with involuntary movements, e.g. athetosis or choreo-athetosis. These movements are not apparent until the 2nd year of life or even later, although the limbs are hypotonic and movement is inco-ordinate. Some cases have associated spasticity.

Speech in these cases is grossly distorted with an explosive dysarthria; there may also be dysphonia or interference with intonation and facial grimacing.

(c) Ataxic

This type is due to involvement of the cerebellar hemispheres and produces various degrees of inco-ordination and hypotonia, often with nystagmus. The speech disorder is due to an ataxic dysarthria.

Various combinations of the above clinical types occur, as well as associated defects, e.g. deafness (which occurs in about 25% of cases, most commonly in the athetoid group), strabismus or other visual defects.

The age at which the diagnosis is made depends upon the severity of the condition, but it is usually within the first 12 to 18 months of life; in others, delay and difficulty in walking are not apparent until later in the 2nd year. The diagnosis of mental defect in early life, depending as it does on failure to achieve new milestones of intellectual development at the normal age (e.g. smiling, following a light, groping for objects, forming syllables and words, etc.) requires experience because of normal variations.

Although a large proportion of patients with cerebral palsy are mentally defective, this is not invariable since gross neurological (e.g. motor) deficits can occur with little or no impairment of mental or intellectual processes. Furthermore, some children with cerebral palsy have specific defects of motor function (apraxia), of sensory function (agnosia), of the special senses (e.g. nerve deafness) or of speech and language ('aphasia', articulatory apraxia, dyslexia—see Chapter 16); these can give a false impression of mental defect if clinical appraisal is superficial or limited. Thus specific defects of speech and other language functions are sometimes misdiagnosed as mental deficiency. However if there is a discrepancy between basic intelligence and language function due to defects predominantly in the sphere of speech and language, then attempts should be made to compensate for the specific disorder by special methods of individual training either of the defective function or of the unaffected functions. It is very important that these children, as well as those with specific non-language disorders (as above), are recognised and educated appropriately; although requiring patient individual training, many can be helped considerably.

In some cases, motor disorders can be alleviated by surgical methods, so helping these children to lead useful lives, but the prognosis will be poor if there are severe intellectual and motor deficits.

INFANTILE HEMIPLEGIA

Infantile hemiplegia can be present from birth (congenital hemiplegia) when it may be due to a cystic deformity of one cerebral hemisphere (porencephaly) or to infarction of the brain occurring in utero. More commonly it develops acutely in infancy or early childhood, often during the course of an acute infection such as whooping cough or following a 'febrile convulsion'. Probably the most common cause is cerebral infarction from arterial or venous occlusion, resulting in scarring and atrophy of the cerebral hemisphere with localised dilatation of the lateral ventricle.

The affected arm is severely paralysed, finger and hand movements being abolished and the hand and forearm assume a typically flexed posture lying across the front of the chest. The leg, though spastic with exaggerated deep reflexes and an extensor plantar response, is less severely affected and all patients are eventually able to walk, often with surprisingly little difficulty.

When bilateral (double hemiplegia) it can be distinguished from the spastic diplegia or cerebral palsy (Little's disease) by the fact that the upper limbs are more severely affected than the lower.

If the dominant hemisphere is involved after speech has developed, aphasia results; the earlier the age of the child the more complete and rapid is the recovery of speech function. If the dominant hemisphere is involved before speech is acquired, the development of speech may be delayed; and in some cases speech function becomes established in the opposite hemisphere.

Residual neurological deficits can be of all grades of severity, but are sometimes only trivial. In the more severe cases, epilepsy is a common complication as the scar in the affected hemisphere acts as a focus of epileptic discharge. In those cases in which epileptic seizures are frequent and severe, brain damage is marked and intellectual impairment and behaviour disorders are common.

CHAPTER 15

DEAFNESS

The development of normal speech is largely dependent on the ability to hear and deafness, if congenital or acquired in infancy, will delay or prevent normal speech development. In any speech disorder of childhood, it is essential to ascertain whether or not there is any hearing defect.

Hearing is the reception of sound by the ear and should be distinguished from listening which is the act of paying attention to what is heard with the object of interpreting its meaning.

The cochlear system is fully developed by twelve weeks of intra-uterine life, although much of the auditory system develops after birth. Although in the new born, hearing produces reflex activity, it does not become discriminatory until about nine months of age.

There are two types of deafness; *perceptive*—where there is a lesion of the auditory nerve or inner ear, and *conductive*—when there is a disorder of the middle ear. Deafness is of the conductive type with no abnormality of the auditory nerve in about 40% of cases. Inner ear or perceptive deafness can be helped by means of a hearing aid because the loudness of the sound reaching the inner ear can be amplified. Patients with conductive deafness sometimes hear better in noisy surroundings and may speak more softly; those with perceptive deafness tend to confuse speech sounds and speak louder than necessary.

A tuning fork will be heard better by bone conduction than air conduction in conductive deafness, as opposed to a normal person who will hear it better by air conduction; a patient with perceptive deafness may not hear by bone conduction at all. To be certain of the amount of deafness a quantitative test of hearing such as pure tone audiometry is necessary.

DEAFNESS IN CHILDREN

The incidence of deafness in children, viz. children requiring deaf education is 1·3/1,000. From the point of view of speech development the age of onset is important. Prior to the advent of anti-biotics, otitis media was the commonest cause of conductive deafness in a school child, although it can also result from eustachian catarrh or just wax in the external meatus. Nerve deafness is an occasional complication of meningitis or mumps in childhood. The various causes are shown in the following classification:

TABLE 12. The aetiology of deafness in children.

PRE-NATAL

1. Agenesis
   (a) cochlear—familial (with abnormalities of pigmentation = Waardenburg syndrome).
   (b) meatal (with failure of facial development = Treacher-Collins syndrome).
2. Infections e.g. rubella, toxoplasmosis, syphilis.
3. Drugs e.g. quinine, thalidomide.
4. Endocrine e.g. cretinism.

PERI-NATAL

1. Birth injury.
2. Anoxia.
3. Prematurity.
4. Kernicterus.

POST-NATAL

Causing perceptive deafness:
1. Infections e.g. meningitis, measles, mumps (which may cause unilateral deafness).
2. Drugs e.g. streptomycin, kanomycin, neomycin.
3. Head injury.

Causing conductive deafness:
4. Chronic suppurative otitis media.
5. Enlarged tonsils and adenoids.

The onset of deafness after speech has developed does not usually interfere with the ability to speak, except that some will tend to shout owing to difficulty gauging the loudness of their voice. Those with deafness due to otosclerosis (usually familial) tend to speak more quietly than normal. Obviously communication will become more difficult as deafness increases, although in some cases a hearing aid may help. Eventually lip-reading and sign language may be necessary. If a deaf person becomes dysphasic, the deafness will obviously add to the problems of speech therapy.

Deafness resulting from disorders of the peripheral hearing mechanism (i.e. the ear and auditory nerve) must be distinguished from difficulty with comprehension due to receptive dysphasia and mental defects. It is very important that there should be no confusion regarding terms such as word-deafness, cortical-deafness and auditory imperception, which describe disabilities of cerebral origin and need different consideration from the usual meaning of deafness, which implies an impairment of the acuity of hearing due to a disorder affecting the peripheral hearing mechanism.

CHAPTER 16

DEVELOPMENTAL SPEECH AND LANGUAGE DISORDERS

The development of a function depends upon learning processes which necessitate not only the making of new physiological pathways but also the inhibition of irrelevant responses, both at physiological and psychological levels. Learning to read and write involves organising a wide variety of perceptual experiences and motor responses, which may be interfered with by bodily disturbances or brain lesions. In the case of language function, the child has to learn to use these skills for the expression of his own feelings. The learning process is not solely dependent on the acquisition of motor skills and perceptual patterns but also on the structuring of the inner world of the child's mind, which is not a 'tabula rasa' but a seething mass of contradictory forces and fantasies, which he must also learn to inhibit when inappropriate. For this reason, it is not surprising that the difficulties of learning methods of communication are often associated with emotional disorders.

A speech defect is a deviation which attracts attention or affects adversely either the speaker or listener. About 10% of children have a speech defect but the incidence becomes less in later age groups. From the age of 6 to 10, 15% are affected but from 10 to 14, this decreases to 5%.

The commonest speech defects in childhood are dyslalia and stammering. Less than 10% of the speech defects are due to cerebral palsy and only 1% due to a cleft palate. Ten percent of the defects are in the nature of dysphasia and only 1% are due to dsyphonia.

Speech disorders in children may be due to temporary or permanent interruptions in the normal development of speech. The majority of children begin to use single words when a year old but the range of normality is wide stretching from 8 months to 2½ years. Words are put together in phrases at about 18 months, again with a wide range from 10 months to $3\frac{1}{2}$ years. In most children, speech is intelligible to the family and friends by the age of 2, but one child in three passes through a phase of unintelligible speech during the third and fourth years. Development does not take place at a steady rate; words are used and lost again and there are often silent periods when little progress is made.

The development of speech depends upon hearing and linking of the sounds and symbols of the spoken word. Poor speech development may result from disorders of 'hearing', 'language', or 'articulation' and many children have multiple disabilities.

The development of speech should be regarded as abnormally delayed if the child is not speaking by the age of $3\frac{1}{2}$ years old. If deafness can be excluded (see Chapter 15) the commonest cause of delayed development of speech is mental defect. Information regarding this can be gathered from the child's other milestones, e.g.

holding head up—three months.
sitting —six months.
standing —nine months.
walking —twelve months.

Other milestones include feeding himself, being clean and dry, ability to dress, playing alone and character of play.

There may be psychological or emotional causes of delayed speech, and a deprived child may not have the stimulus to speak e.g. because of being in an institution. With all speech disorders, boys are more commonly affected than girls, and this is particularly so in stammering (see Chapter 17).

The importance of cerebral dominance is controversial in developmental speech disorders but left-handedness and ambidexterity appear commoner both in affected children and their relatives; in one series, 5% of normal children were left-handed whereas 50% of the affected children showed signs of cerebral ambilaterally i.e. mixed dominance with a combination of, say, left-handedness and right-eyedness. The failure to establish a completely dominant hemisphere is not necessarily the cause of the delayed speech but may be an associated abnormality of brain function.

CLASSIFICATION:

The diagnosis of disorders of speech and language in children can be one of inordinate complexity. Not only does it involve many disciplines but the decision as to whether speech is delayed for pathological reasons can also be difficult. These can be classified into disorders:

1. of articulation
   (a) neurological (see Chapters 6 and 7).
   (b) mechanical (e.g. hare-lip).
   (c) dyslalia.
2. of voice—dysphonia (see Chapter 8).
3. of language—developmental dysphasia.
4. of reading and writing—developmental dyslexia and dysgraphia.
5. of rhythm—chiefly stammering (see Chapter 17).
6. secondary to
   (a) deafness—central and peripheral (see Chapter 15).
   (b) mental factors—amentia or subnormality.
   (c) psychiatric factors (autism, elective mutism).
   (d) environmental factors (lack of stimulus).

Dyslalia is the immature pronunciation of words, for which there is no obvious structural cause. This is the commonest cause of referral to speech therapists in school clinics.

Children over the age of 5 with immature patterns of speech (e.g. speech may be like that of a three year old) may lisp, e.g. have rhoticism where there is difficulty with 'r' or sigmatism where there is difficulty with 's'. These immature forms of speech are grouped together as 'dyslalia'. There is no defect in the nervous system apart from the continuing immature speech—lips, tongue and palate move normally when tested and there is no apraxic difficulty so that there is normally a rapid response to appropriate treatment, e.g. practising the proper pronunciation of words under supervision. Dyslalia must be differentiated from articulatory dyspraxia (apraxic dysarthria) in which children are unable to imitate speech sounds, so that their response to treatment is much less satisfactory. Dyslalia must also be differentiated from the other forms of 'lalling' or idioglossia.

Developmental dysphasia:

There are nearly thirty synonyms, e.g. auditory agnosia, congenital auditory perception, subcortical central deafness, idiopathic language retardation, alalia, aphemia, audimutitas, word deafness, minimal cerebral impairment. Many of these terms suggest an aetiological cause or anatomical substrate which has not yet been proven.

The terms congenital or developmental dysphasia are paradoxical in that dysphasia—as strictly defined—is the loss of the ability to express or understand speech after it has been acquired; this differs from defects of speech which have not been fully developed. The same sort of difference exists between dementia (which is the loss or disintegration of the established mental functions) and amentia (which is the failure of development of mental functions).

Like adult aphasia, the speech defect may be mainly on the expressive side, i.e. these children can understand most of what is said especially if it is spoken slowly, but in the more severe cases they cannot. The failure to speak in these cases is often compensated for by gesture.

The case histories of children with developmental dysphasia can be divided into two groups. In the first, so-called 'developmental' or 'congenital' aphasia, there is often a history of birth trauma as evidenced by difficult labour, breech delivery, twin pregnancy, forceps or precipitate delivery and prematurity. Babble is not well developed and this is a significant feature since other milestones may be normal.

The second group is 'acquired' aphasia. These children develop speech normally, i.e. prelinguistic babble is normal and, depending on the age of onset, two word phrases and sentences are spoken. Between the ages of 2½ and 6, during a period of days or a few weeks, hearing appears to be lost and then speech goes, perhaps with a stammer, so that within a short time these children may become completely aphasic. Epileptic attacks may occur at, or soon after, the onset. Although tumours etc. have to be excluded, investigations such as X-rays of the skull, lumbar puncture, air encephalography and carotid arteriography are almost invariably normal. The electroencephalogram (E.E.G.) is usually abnormal especially over the temporal area on the dominant side; these E.E.G. abnormalities, like the fits, subside spontaneously over the ensuing few months or years.

Another clinical difference between the 'developmental' and 'acquired' groups is the sex incidence. The developmental cases, like those with specific dyslexia and stammerers are more commonly boys but the acquired group shows no predilection for either sex.

As would be expected, the acquired cases show psychiatric disturbances e.g. temper-tantrums, mood changes and alteration in personality which may mistakenly suggest a psychogenic aetiology. These are not so common in the congenital group.

The diagnosis is made difficult by the variable responses to sound e.g. these children will respond to their names at some times but not at others. Audiometry often shows a loss in the high frequency ranges which improves over the years—whether to conditioning or 'maturation' is uncertain. Evoked potentials with noise using E.E.G. recordings during sleep and evoked response audiometry reveal responses in the auditory areas proving that peripheral deafness is not the primary disturbance.

Routine neurological examination of both these groups is usually negative, i.e. very rarely are 'hard' signs such as brisk reflexes or extensor plantar responses found but there is evidence of 'soft' signs of motor dysfunction if measured by the Lincoln-Osaretsky test. For this reason these children are thought to have 'minimal brain damage'.

Even in the absence of neurological signs there can be little doubt that the cause is physiogenic (cf. migraine, epilepsy), but it is difficult to state 'where' and 'what' the lesion is. The localisation of a lesion is not the same as the localisation of a function and attempts to understand children's speech disturbances by analogies with adult lesions may be deceptive and unjustifiable. However the anatomical site of the defect is possibly the inferior parietal lobule (supramarginal and angular gyri, Brodmann's areas 39 & 40). This is the 'association area of association areas' upon which projection fibres from the primary motor, sensory, visual and auditory areas impinge. This area is particularly important since speech depends on the ability to form cross-modal associations. The inferior parietal lobule is unique to man (as is speech) and like all recent evolutionary areas in the brain, myelinates late and also shows late dendrogenesis (formation of dendrites). It is possible to speculate that the rapidly growing and 'maturing' area is peculiarly sensitive to noxious stimuli and produces the 'disconnection syndrome' of developmental aphasia.

Developmental (specific) dyslexia:
A difference of at least two years between mental and reading ages is probably outside normal limits and the term specific or developmental dyslexia is used; because the range of normality is so wide some educationalists have doubted the existence of specific dyslexia.

The commonest cause of backwardness in reading is subnormal intelligence with diminution of the overall learning ability. In borderline cases formal assessment of the intelligence quotient by psychological testing is helpful. In some children difficulties arise because they are distractable and restless with poor attention span. This may be due to the syndrome of 'chronic minimal brain damage', which is manifest as backwardness in reading, writing, speaking or clumsy movements quite apart from behaviour disorders, often with a hyperkinetic state. Milestones may be normal but, if delayed, can give an indication of brain damage and there may be corroborative evidence in the history. On psychological testing visuo-spatial abnormalities are often found so that there is reversal or transposition of letters at a later age than normal.

There is often an inconsistency in the mistakes, the child at one time being able to read or write a letter or word but not at another time. These children are often able to mirror-write and mirror-read. Reading and writing of letters are often much better than of words.

Other causes of difficulty in learning to read must be excluded e.g. visual defect, poor teaching (large classes or poor school attendance) and difficulty in home circumstances. Another cause is an emotional block (said to be the cause in the difficulty in reading of Hans Christian Andersen).

The age incidence of diagnosis is between 6 to 9 years. Boys suffer from this far more commonly than girls in the proportion of 5 to 1. Hallgren gave a rough estimate of the incidence of specific dyslexia as 10%. There is often a history of twinning in the family with concordance in monozygotic twins and discordance in 2/3 of dizygotic twins. There is often a family history of dyslexia and there may be an increased incidence of left-handedness in relatives. The significance of left-handedness depends on the criteria used for testing hand dominance. The various difficulties in reading consist of:

(1) inability to work out the pronunciation of a strange word,
(2) failure to see likeness and differences in forms of words,
(3) failure to see differences in shapes of letters,
(4) making reversals,
(5) failure to keep the place,
(6) failure to read from left to right,
(7) poor concentration,
(8) failure to read with sufficient understanding.

TABLE 13. Examination of developmental disorders of speech in children.

The following table shows the main headings for a simple clinical assessment of speech defects in children. Tests must of course be geared to the age of the child and it should be emphasised that a complete and accurate assessment needs a multidisciplinary team which would include an educational psychologist and audiologist as well as a speech therapist.

A. Receptive:
(1) Auditory acuity.
(2) Reaction to sounds.
(3) Speech comprehension with face seen.
(4) Speech comprehension with face unseen.
(5) Comprehending pantomime.

B. Expressive:
(1) Noises.
(2) Words.
(3) Pantomime.

C. Reading:

D. Writing:

E. Cerebral dominance:

F. General behaviour:
(1) Interaction with other people.
(2) Interaction with animals, objects, tests.

The commonest difficulties found are confusion of letters which have a visual resemblance, such as 'p' and 'q', 'b' and 'd'. More often a child can read the individual letters but makes mistakes with them when reading words. The mistakes made in reading do not differ from those made by a normal child learning to read. The reading speed is reduced and, in addition, the understanding of what has been read is also reduced.

There are often associated writing disabilities viz. confusion or disfigurement of letters, errors in linking together letters with contamination, mirror-writing, block letters and reversals.

These children may also have disorders of motility, for example (1) dyspraxia, (2) minor sensory disorders, (3) inadequate directional motions, (4) right-to-left confusion with alterations in body image and simultanagnosia and possibly (5) a faulty estimation of time. Aetiological explanations include:

(1) a specific lesion near the angular gyrus,
(2) delayed maturation in the parieto-occipital area,
(3) disturbed Gestalt function,
(4) lack of cerebral dominance.

CHAPTER 17

STAMMERING

There is a vast literature, but little agreement, on the causation of stammering. From one centre alone up to 1955, there were 153 dissertations and 255 publications and in the past 10 years the number of reports from all over the world make an analysis of the findings difficult. The main area of dispute is whether stammering is simply an expression of neurosis ('the psychogenic' theory), or whether it has an organic basis, (the 'physiogenic' theory) or whether it is due to a combination of both. There is no doubt that anxiety states occur in many stammerers but whether they are primary or secondary is controversial.

Nomenclature is made difficult because of the use of other terms. Stuttering is the term more commonly used in the United States and some authorities suggest that it is a more severe form of stammering or has a different aetiological background. The two terms are here considered as synonymous.

Definition

Stammering is a deviation of speech which attracts attention or affects adversely the speaker or listener because of an interruption in the normal rhythm of speech by involuntary repetition, prolongation or arrest of sounds. This does not take into account the unreliable judgement of listener or speaker—what is stammering to one person is not necessarily so to another; one speaker may consider that he is stammering when he is not and vice versa. During the development of speech, most children repeat syllables and words (echolalia), and some normal adults stammer under emotional stress. Estimates have been made of the number of repetitions in normal speech; in normal children between the ages of two and five years old there is a repetition of words, syllables or phrases about 45 times in every 1,000 running words, the upper limit being 100 times per 1,000 running words. More than this produces a noticeable stammer.

Incidence

This depends on the age of the series investigated. In children of school age estimates have varied from 0·7% to 4% whereas in adults the incidence is 0·5%. This means that there are about a quarter of a million stammerers in this country and over 15 million stammerers in the world.

Age of onset

Eighty-five percent of stammerers begin to do so before the age of 8; there are probably two peaks, namely at about 2–3 years, when the child starts to speak and 6–8 years when the child learns to read soon after starting school and mixing with other children; the incidence certainly decreases by the age of 10 years.

Sex incidence

Like speech defects in general, it is commoner in boys; the exact proportion, like its frequency, varies with age. Stammering tends to persist more with boys so that the discrepancy of incidence in the two sexes increases with age. Under the age of 6 years there are twice as many boys as girls affected whilst at all ages there are probably seven times as many males as females affected.

Genetic factors

There is a familial incidence of stammering varying in different series from 36% to 65%. These estimates vary because of the differences in defining a stammerer and the type of relatives included, e.g. whether only first degree relatives (or also cousins, uncles and grandparents as well as parents and siblings). The familial incidence does not necessarily imply a genetic factor since environmental factors could also apply to more than one member of the family and, since mimicry is one of the modes of learning in children, imitation is a powerful factor. In families with stammerers, twins are more likely to stammer than the other children. Stammering is more common in identical than non-identical twins but, in these cases, the sex incidence does not show the usual male preponderance. Interestingly, the incidence of stammering is greater in families in which twinning occurs than in families without twins.

Stammering occurs more frequently with consonants than vowels in the proportion of about 5 to 1; the vast majority of stammering incidents (96 %) are associated with the initial sounds of the word.

Factors that improve stammering are:

(1) speaking in unison (2) modifying the voice by singing, whispering, acting or using a different pitch (3) repetition of rhymes, stories and choral speaking.

Aggravating factors include emotional states such as anxiety and anger (although this latter sometimes improves it), rapid speech, answering questions and speaking to superiors.

Experimentally, it has been shown that people with normal speech may have their speech disturbed by delayed playback speech, i.e. playing a tape record back through well fitting headphones with speech delayed 1/10 to 1/5 sec. With this there is an excessive drawling of vowels with word repetition and stammering. This suggests that the production of speech involves a closed-cycle feed-back by which means a speaker continually monitors and checks his own voice production. Stammering can be almost totally inhibited by interfering with a stammerer's perceptions suggesting that the determining defects are perceptual rather than motor. Auditory perception may be interfered with by deafness or by compelling transference of the speaker's perceptions to a source of sound other than his own speech. Stammering is less common in deaf children.

Shadowing, i.e. copying the speech of another person, is an imitative motor action which often abolishes stammer, presumably because the subjects perception is transferred away from his own voice to the control speaker's voice. Some stammerers have no speech difficulty when singing in a choir or reciting in unison—this is not the same as shadowing because the stimulus is learned. In simultaneous reading, the control could change the text, or even speak gibberish and yet the stammerer continues to read the original text without stammering; this suggests it is not words or the interpretation of semantic concept which exercises control over the stammerer but the sounds themselves, or some elements of the sounds, which may simply act as a distraction.

When a person hears his own voice he hears it by bone and air conduction whereas, in shadowing, he hears it only by air conduction. These pathways differ in their acoustic properties. The stimuli are comparable in loudness but there is a difference in the pitch of sounds transmitted (cf. listening to one's own recorded voice where we hear our own speaking voices at a higher pitch because bone-conducted sounds manifest a low frequency emphasis).

Cerebral dominance

Estimates of sinistrality amongst stammerers vary because of differences in testing handedness and footedness etc. In one series, 11% were left handed and 5% left sided, as opposed to 6% and 3% respectively in controls.

Earlier reports suggested that the majority of stammerers were cases of shifted sinistrality but this has not been generally confirmed.

Left-handedness is commoner in twins, 10% being sinistrals as opposed to the expected 4%. Over 5% of twins stammer which is more than five times the expected number, and it has been suggested that there was a genetic link between twinning, stammering and sinistrality. Electroencephalography in some cases shows that the alpha rhythm is more symmetrical in stammerers (normally the alpha waves are of lower voltage on the dominant side); this suggests less complete dominance but there is no statistical difference between stammerers and normals.

Imperfect lateralisation for speech indicates lack of cerebral dominance (cerebral ambilaterality) and although this does not imply any psychological abnormality the 'possessor of this type of cerebral organisation is particularly vulnerable to the effects of stress' (Zangwill 1960). In the ambilateral, the proper development of reading and writing, spatial judgement and directional control is relatively easily disturbed e.g. by brain injury at birth, or problems in psychological adjustment. A bilingual upbringing, for example, is often noted in stammerers and may be a significant factor in some cases.

It seems likely that there is a constitutional predisposition together with environmental factors as the basis of the multifactorial aetiology of stammering.

SELECTED BIBLIOGRAPHY

Chapter 1

BRAIN LORD (1965) *Speech Disorders* 2nd Ed. Butterworths. London

MASON S.E. (1963) *Signs, Signals and Symbols* Methuen. London

Chapter 2

BOWSHER D. (1967) *Introduction to the Anatomy and Physiology of the Nervous System* Blackwell. Oxford

BREWER C.V. (1961) *The Organisation of the Central Nervous System* Heinemann. London

CARTERETTE E.C. (1966) *Brain Function: Speech, Language and Communication* University of California Press. Los Angeles

CHERRY C. (1961) *On Human Communication* John Wiley & Sons. New York

MILLIKAN C.H. & DARLEY F.L. (1967) *Brain Mechanisms Underlying Speech and Language* Grune & Stratton. London

NATHAN P. (1969) *The Nervous System* Penguin. London

ROSE F.C. & SYMONDS C.P. (1960) Organic memory loss following encephalitis *Brain*, **83**, 195

RUSSELL W.R. (1959) *Brain, Memory, Learning* Clarendon Press. Oxford

RUSSELL W.R. (1963) Some anatomical aspects of aphasia *Lancet*, **1**, 1173

Chapter 3

CRITCHLEY M. (1953) *The Parietal Lobes* Arnold. London

Chapter 4

HÉCAEN H. & AJURIAGUERRA J. (1964) *Left Handedness* Grune & Stratton. London

MILNER B., BRANCH C. & RASMUSSEN T. (1964) *Disorders of Language* Ed. by deReuck A.V.S. & O'Connor M. Churchill. London

PENFIELD W. & ROBERTS L. (1959) *Speech and Brain Mechanisms* Oxford University Press. London

RUSSELL W.R. & ESPIR M.L.E. (1961) *Traumatic Aphasia* Oxford University Press. London

ZANGWILL O.L. (1960) *Cerebral Dominance and its Relation to Psychological Function* Oliver and Boyd. Edinburgh

Chapter 5

CRITCHLEY M. (1970) *Aphasiology* Arnold. London

RIOCH D.M. & WEINSTEIN E.A. (1964) *Disorders of Communication* Williams & Wilkins. Baltimore

SCHUELL H., JENKINS J.J. & JIMENEZ-PABON E. (1964) *Aphasia in Adults* Harper and Row. New York

WEPMAN J.M. (1951) *Recovery fr om Aphasia* Ronald Press Co. New York

WILLIS, T. (1683) *Two Discourses Concerning the Soul of Brutes* Pordage. London

Chapter 6

BICKERSTAFF E.R. (1965) *Neurology for Nurses* English Universities Press. London

Chapter 7

WALTON J.N. (1961) *Essentials of Neurology* Pitman. London

Chapter 8

DRAPER I.T. (1968) *Lecture Notes on Neurology* 2nd Ed. Blackwell. Oxford

Chapter 9

BROMLEY D.B. (1966) *The Psychology of Human Ageing* Penguin. London

EYSENCK A.J. (1962) *Know Your Own I.Q.* Penguin. London

GATHERCOLE C.E. (1968) *Assessment in Clinical Psychology* Penguin. London

TERWILLIGER R.F. (1968) *Meaning and Mind: a Study in the Psychology of Language* Oxford University Press. London

ZANGWILL O. (1943) *Proc. roy. Soc. med.* **35**, 36

Chapter 10

FAIRFIELD L. (1954) *Epilepsy* Gerald Duckworth. London

SUTHERLAND J.M. & TAIT H. (1969) *The Epilepsies* Livingstone. Edinburgh & London

Chapter 11

OLIVER L. (1969) *Removable Intracranial Tumours* Heinemann. London

Chapter 12

MARSHALL J. (1968) *The Management of Cerebro-vascular Disease* 2nd Ed. Churchill. London

MATTHEWS W.B. (1963) *Practical Neurology* Blackwell. Oxford

Chapter 13

BRAIN, LORD & WALTON J. (1969) *Diseases of the Nervous System* Medical Publications. Oxford

Chapter 14

CARTER C.O. (1962) *Human Heredity* Penguin. London

LAING J. (1968) *Assessment of the Cerebral Palsied Child for Education* Heinemann. Spastics Society

MECHAM M.J., BERKO M.J. & BERKO F.G. (1960) *Speech Therapy in Cerebral Palsy* Charles C. Thomas. Springfield, Ill

ROBERTS J.A.F. (1959) *An Introduction to Medical Genetics* Oxford University Press. London

Chapter 15

WHETNALL E. & FRY D.B. (1964) *The Deaf Child* Heinemann. London

Chapter 16

CRITCHLEY M. (1969) *The Dyslexic Child* 2nd Ed. Heinemann. London

FLOW R.M., GOFMAN H.F. & LAWSON L.I. (1965) *Reading Disorders* F.A. Davis Co. Philadelphia Pa.

FRANKLIN A.W. (1962) *Word Blindness or Specific Developmental Dyslexia* Pitman. London

FRANKLIN A.W. (1965) *Children with Communication Problems* Pitman. London

HALLGREN B. (1950) Specific dyslexia *Acta. Psych. Neurol.* Suppl. 65

INGRAM T.T.S. (1969) Disorders of speech in childhood *Brit. J. hosp. Med.* **10** 1608

RENFREW C. & MURPHY K. (1964) *The Child who does not Talk* Heinemann. London

Chapter 17

ANDREWS G. & HARRIS M. (1964) *The Syndrome of Stuttering* Heinemann. London

JOHNSON W. (1961) *Stuttering* University of Minnesota Press. Minneapolis

INDEX